CANCER

A Biological and Clinical Introduction

Second Edition

Steven B. Oppenheimer

California State University,
Northridge

Jones and Bartlett Publishers, Inc.
Boston/Portola Valley

Medicine, to produce health, has to examine disease.

Plutarch
Lives, Demetrius

To the American Cancer Society and dedicated students and faculty who have brought us programs in the biology of cancer, *and* to the National Cancer Institute and National Science Foundation for research support.

Cover photo: Scanning electron micrograph of dividing cells. From G. Shih and R. Kessel. 1982. *Living Images.* Jones and Bartlett Publishers, Inc.

Editorial offices: Jones and Bartlett Publishers, Inc., 30 Granada Court, Portola Valley, CA 94025

Sales and customer service offices: Jones and Bartlett Publishers, Inc., 20 Park Plaza, Boston, MA 02116

Library of Congress Cataloging in Publication Data
Oppenheimer, Steven B., 1944–
   Cancer, a biological and clinical introduction.

   Includes bibliographies and index.
   1. Cancer. I. Title. [DNLM: 1. Neoplasms.
QZ 200 064c]
RC261.064   1984   616.99'407   85-18182
ISBN 0-86720-062-6

Design/Production: Unicorn Production Services
Printer/Binder: Alpine Press

Printed in the United States of America
10 9 8 7 6 5 4 3 2 1

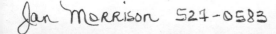

Preface to the Second Edition

Rapid advances in certain aspects of cancer biology, in particular, the study of oncogenes, have made it necessary to update the first edition of this book one or two years earlier than originally planned. A great deal of enthusiasm from teachers and students who have used the book in the past two years has given me the interest to prepare this revision.

The book has been updated, a new chapter on oncogenes has been added, and most of the figures have been redrawn. Furthermore, the text has been revised and clarified, a task guided by David Freifelder, and read by Rachel Freifelder, both of whom deserve my thanks.

The instructor and students will note that many concepts and facts appear numerous times in the book, frequently duplicating what has been presented before. This pedagogical device has been considered advisable in view of the complexity of the topic and the variability in backgrounds of the students.

I appreciate the enthusiasm of Arthur Bartlett, who agreed to include the book in the Jones and Bartlett publishing program, and the administration of Allyn and Bacon who allowed the transfer of copyright in order that the second edition could be published rapidly.

Steven B. Oppenheimer
August, 1985

Preface to the
First Edition

In recent years, courses in the biology of cancer have found a place in the curricula of numerous undergraduate institutions and health-related, professional programs. Having been associated with such a course, sponsored by the American Cancer Society, I have become keenly aware of the need for a text in this area that treats both cellular aspects of cancer and the clinical aspects of the disease in an organized, clear, and coherent manner. It is hoped that this text will provide a balanced treatment of the entire cancer problem that is stimulating and clearly presented for undergraduates, nurses, and other health professionals.

The text begins with the cellular aspects of cancer and concludes with the clinical and organismal aspects of the disease. What causes cancer? What causes cancer to spread? What are the characteristics of cancer cells? Can our body defenses attack cancer cells? What are the similarities and differences between different tumors? What is the intriguing relationship between cancer cells and embryo cells? Is cancer inherited? Is cancer infectious? How is it diagnosed? How is it treated? What are some new experimental methods of cancer treatment?

These are some of the questions that are examined in this text. Not all of the answers to these sorts of questions are at hand but some are. It is hoped that this text will provide the reader with some of the answers and with an understanding of the ways in which investigators approach the study of cancer. Also, I hope that sharing my own enthusiasm for the subject matter will excite the curiosity and interest of students so that some may eventually contribute to the body of knowledge concerning one of the most dreaded diseases.

I wish to thank Michael Edidin, Heinrich Ursprung, Malcolm Steinberg, Saul Roseman, Stephen Roth, and Robert DeHaan, who served as the nucleus of individuals at Johns Hopkins who helped provide me with the foundations needed to write this text. I would also like to express my gratitude to the National Cancer Institute, the American Cancer Society, and the National Science Foundation for supporting my research efforts and my program in cancer biology at Northridge.

Special thanks is given to Joseph Burns, Editor, Allyn and Bacon, who skillfully steered this book through all of the phases of its development. He has not been just an editor but has actively participated in molding content and style. I thank Gary Folven, Managing Editor, who has helped me over the years by providing an excellent atmosphere in which to work. I thank Judith Gimple and Sarah Doyle of Bywater Production Services for a meticulous job and the entire staff at Allyn and Bacon for their enthusiastic assistance.

I would like to thank all my colleagues who have kindly provided photos and permission to use illustrations of their work in this book. I am particularly indebted to the American Cancer Society, Robert Dyson, David Epel, Harvey Gilbert, Garth Nicolson, Nuclear Associates, R. E. Saxton, K. Tanaka, Victor Vacquier, and Varian Associates for providing collections of superb micrographs and charts.

I would like to make special mention and express my gratitude to the many fine reviewers who have helped guide me in the writing of this book: Peter B. Armstrong, University of California, Davis; Lois M. Bergquist, Los Angeles Valley College; Joel S. Greenberger, Harvard Medical School; Charles M. Haskell, Wadsworth Cancer Center; George Lefevre; California State University, Northridge; George M. Malacinski, Indiana University; Robert G. McKinnell; University of Minnesota; Richard Schwarz, University of California, Berkeley; John R. Seffrin; Indiana University; Rachel Spector, Boston College; Michelle Stuart, Rush Presbyterian-St. Luke's Hospital; Robert A. Weinberg, Massachusetts Institute of Technology; and Melanie Wolf, Houston, Texas. I have taken much of the advice of these reviewers. Any errors, however, are my own. Finally, I wish to thank my wife Carolyn for excellent typing and suggestions and a superb sense of humor.

Steven B. Oppenheimer
1982

Contents

12

Diagnosis of Cancer   159

13

Treatments for Cancer   173

14

Protection Against Cancer   199

15

Psychosocial Aspects of Cancer   213

16

The Prognosis for Cancer   223

1

Introduction

Diseases such as plague, smallpox, polio, and diphtheria were once major scourges of the world. However, in the past few decades, with the introduction of antibiotics and vaccines, the incidence and seriousness of infectious diseases has become minor. Now, the diseases that usually affect older individuals, namely, heart disease, stroke, and cancer, which account for 37.8, 20.4, and 9.6 percent, respectively, of all deaths in the United States, are the major causes of death; and a major effort is in progress to combat these diseases. Heart disease and stroke are usually progressive and not totally curable; however, many cancers have become curable to some extent (Tables 1-1, 1-2). After reading this book, students should feel generally optimistic that the incidence of death by cancer will continue to fall in the future. Although the current statistics of cancer incidence and mortality appear grim, numerous specific cancers, such as acute leukemia in children, which once was considered incurable, today is curable in an increasing number of cases.

The relation between survival rates and death rates, and the expectation for changes in these values, has in the past primarily reflected new treatments. However, these values do not really indicate what can be expected in the future, because they do not indicate possible changes caused by reducing the incidence of cancer. For example; one of the major cancer killers, lung cancer, is seldom diagnosed early enough to effect a cure, and indeed death rates from

TABLE 1-1 Progress against cancer

Period	Fraction alive after 5 years
1930s	Less than 1 in 5
1950s	Less than 1 in 4
1970s	1 in 3

TABLE 1-2 5-year survival rates for certain cancers

Site	Condition of tumor at time of detection	
	Localized	Spread
Bladder	72%	14%
Breast	85	47
Colon-rectum	71	26
Larynx	79	32
Lung	33	4
Oral	67	25
Prostate	70	35
Uterus-cervix	78	37

lung cancer are increasing (Tables 1-3, 1-4). However, lung cancer is largely preventable. Eighty percent of the roughly 100,000 new lung cancer patients detected annually are smokers, and many of the other patients are workers in high-risk occupations, such as those dealing with specific carcinogenic substances like asbestos. Lung cancer deaths in the United States are about a third of the total number of deaths from all other kinds of cancers combined. Elimination of smoking may in time reduce cancer death rates by 50 percent! Smoking is also believed to be a major cause of numerous other types of cancers, and these too would be reduced by the elimination (or at least substantial reduction) of smoking.

It seems unlikely that smoking will be eliminated in the near future. However, a decline in lung cancer deaths could result from the introduction of cigarettes with reduced amounts of tar and nicotine. A recent study by the American Cancer Society, carried out over a 12-year period with one million individuals, has indicated that the rate of death by lung cancer in users of low-tar and low-nicotine cigarettes was 26 percent lower than that among smokers of standard cigarettes. (This is not to say that these cigarettes are safe, because the death rate due to lung cancer among these smokers is still six times greater than that of the general population.) Thus, progress in reducing lung cancer deaths in the short run must rely in part on the tobacco companies marketing less hazardous cigarettes.

THE PROBLEM OF EARLY DIAGNOSIS

A major reason for the high death rate with some types of cancer is the fact that they are detected fairly late. For example, lung cancer

TABLE 1-3 Summary of cancer death rates, 1930-1976

Men	Women
Substantial decrease	
Stomach (6-fold)	Uterus (4-fold)
	Stomach (7-fold)
About the same	
Colon-rectum	Breast
Prostate	Colon-rectum
Pancreas	Ovary
Esophagus	Lung
Leukemia	Pancreas
Bladder	Leukemia
Substantial increase	
Lung (18-fold)	Lung (4-fold)

TABLE 1-4 25-year trends in cancer death rates per 100,000 population, 1950–1952 to 1975–1977.

Sex	Sites	1950–52	1975–77	Percent changes	Comments
Male	All Sites	131.1	102.3	+ 23.8	Steady increase mainly due to lung cancer.
Female	All Sites	118.9	107.9	− 9.3	Slight decrease.
Male	Bladder	5.1	4.9	*	Slight fluctuations; overall no change.
Female	Bladder	2.2	1.4	− 35.1	Some fluctuations; noticeable decrease.
Male	Breast	0.3	0.3	*	Constant rate.
Female	Breast	22.0	23.2	+ 0.6	Slight fluctuations; overall no change.
Male	Colon & rectum	19.4	19.0	− 2.1	Slight fluctuations; overall no change.
Female	Colon & rectum	18.9	14.9	− 19.5	Slight fluctuations; noticeable decrease.
Male	Esophagus	3.6	4.3	+ 19.0	Some fluctuations; slight increase.
Female	Esophagus	.9	1.2	*	Slight fluctuations; overall no change in females.
Male	Kidney	2.8	3.7	+ 32.1	Steady slight increase.
Female	Kidney	1.6	1.8	*	Slight fluctuations; overall no change.
Male	Leukemia	6.5	6.9	+ 6.2	Early increase, later leveling off.
Female	Leukemia	4.6	4.1	− 8.7	Slight early increase, later leveling off and decrease.
Male	Lung	18.3	56.7	+210.6	Steady increase in both sexes due to cigarette smoking.
Female	Lung	3.9	14.0	+263.3	
Male	Oral	4.7	4.8	*	Slight fluctuations; overall no change in both sexes.
Female	Oral	1.2	1.6	*	
Female	Ovary	7.0	7.3	+ 4.3	Steady increase, later leveling off.
Male	Pancreas	6.5	8.4	+ 29.2	Steady increase in both sexes, then leveling off.
Female	Pancreas	4.2	5.2	+ 23.8	Reasons unknown.
Male	Prostate	13.3	13.9	+ 5.3	Fluctuations all through period; overall no change.
Male	Skin	2.3	2.8	*	Slight fluctuations; overall no change in both sexes.
Female	Skin	1.5	1.6	*	
Male	Stomach	17.6	6.8	− 61.2	Steady decrease in both sexes; reasons unknown.
Female	Stomach	9.3	3.2	− 65.6	
Female	Uterus	18.2	7.4	− 59.3	Steady decrease.

* Percent changes not listed because they are not meaningful.
Source: *Cancer Facts and Figures.* New York: American Cancer Society, 1980.

is usually not diagnosed until the tumor is about 1 cm in diameter, and such a tumor already contains about one billion cells. It has been estimated that many lung cancers require ten years to reach this size, and during this time the cells may have spread to other parts of the body. As shown in Table 1-2 the prognosis (the chances for cure) for a cancer that has spread is much poorer than that for one that has been diagnosed before spreading has occurred. Improved diagnostic techniques that enable a much smaller tumor to be detected should reduce the death rate. Development of such techniques is a feature of the research effort against cancer.

A major success story in decreasing cancer deaths by early diagnosis is that of cancer of the cervix (Tables 1-3, 1-4). The lower death rate due to cervical cancer is almost exclusively a result of the widespread use of the Pap test. In this test a smear of vaginal cells is taken and examined by microscopy. Abnormal cells can be observed, and often precancerous conditions can be identified and treated before spreading occurs.

We face a complex interplay of various factors when discussing cancer death rates and cures. Not only must one be concerned with diagnostic techniques and methods of treatment, but also with public attitudes, habits (for example, to smoke or not), and awareness. Specialists in public health have recognized for some time that improvements in any of these areas will greatly reduce cancer death rates and that education of the public must be given highest priority. Throughout this text, we will see these features of the cancer problem. It goes without saying that combating cancer also requires knowledge of the causes of cancer, as we now understand them. The causes of cancer will be a major part of this book and will be discussed in some detail. However, it is valuable to have a preliminary look at some general aspects of factors that appear to be involved in causing cancer. These are presented briefly in the next section.

CAUSES OF CANCER

From studies of humans and other vertebrates a variety of factors have been implicated in causing cancer. These factors include environmental agents (chemicals, ionizing radiation, ultraviolet radiation), the genetic constitution of the individual, gross chromosomal abnormalities, hormonal dysfunctions, and viruses.

Cancer is a disease in which cells grow in an uncontrolled way. Most cells in the body are neither growing nor dividing, and those that do are strictly controlled. However, cancer cells are not subject to the mechanisms of growth control present in most normal cells, and hence they multiply. As a result of their continual division and spreading, cancer cells eventually interfere with one or more vital functions and cause death. Anything that can interfere with the normal control of cell division may lead to cancer. For more than 200 years it has been recognized that long-term exposure to certain substances increases the probability of cancer. In fact, from accumulated statistics it is now estimated that perhaps 90 percent of all human cancers are caused by exposure to environmental agents. As we will see, these factors include not only manufactured substances but also sunlight and naturally occurring agents in our diets. Substances and agents that cause cancer are called carcinogens.

Chemical studies of many carcinogens have shown that most of these substances act either directly or indirectly on cellular DNA and thereby alter genetic information. In fact, most compounds that cause cancer have also been shown to cause mutations in DNA. For this reason, in the next chapter we will examine the structure of DNA and the mechanism of production of mutations.

Nuclear radiation is an important cause of cancer. This had been suspected for many years but was made clear by determining cancer rates among survivors of the atom bomb blasts in Japan. The rates of many types of leukemia among the exposed population are correlated closely with the radiation exposure. Study of the effects of radiation on a variety of cells (bacteria, animal cells, plant cells) has shown that the primary damage caused by radiation is again to the DNA, both breakage of the molecules and alteration of its informational content.

An important feature of cancer is that frequently a tumor does not develop until a very long time after exposure to a carcinogenic agent, perhaps 20 years. This observation has led to the belief that cancer does not result from a single molecular change in a cell but may require several distinct alterations, each of which may occur at very different times. This hypothesis was made more certain by studies with particular classes of cancer-causing agents that cannot cause cancer by themselves. These classes, called initiators and promoters, have the property that tissue must be exposed to one agent of each class and that exposure need not be simultaneous. In fact, all that is needed is that the initiator be applied first. Exposure to the promoter can occur years after exposure to the initiator. The hypothesis, which will be examined in Chapter 6 is that the first step (initiation) involves a permanent change, such as a mutation, while the second step (promotion) involves some sort of stimulus that causes the initiated cells to divide. The existence of these two classes of substances, specific combinations of which are required for cancer induction, sometimes makes identification of substances that cause cancer quite difficult. For example, a test for the activity of a carcinogen may give a negative result if the appropriate initiator is unknown and thus not used in the test.

The genetic makeup of an individual is definitely important in the development of some cancers. For example, bilateral retinoblastoma, a cancer that develops in the eyes of children, is clearly inherited. An individual receiving the bilateral retinoblastoma gene from a parent will develop the cancer. However, most cancers and precancerous conditions do not appear to be inherited, at least not directly. The predisposition to develop cancer or certain types of cancers may have a genetic basis; however, if so, it is much more complicated than for bilateral retinoblastoma. For example, lung cancer is much more prevalent in smokers who have a close relative with lung cancer than in smokers who do not have such a family history. Such a correlation suggests a predisposition with a genetic basis, but still the actual carcinogens from tobacco smoke are the agents that cause the cancer in these individuals. Some breast cancers and many other cancers also show a tendency to run in families, in that a daughter has a slightly enhanced probability of developing breast cancer if her mother also had breast cancer.

Viruses are also known to cause cancer in animals, for example, leukemia in cats and mice, and sarcomas in chickens. Proof comes from experiments in which isolated viruses are injected into susceptible animals and tumors appear several months later. The evidence for viruses as an agent of cancer in man is less conclusive. The herpes viruses appear to be associated with some human cancers, such as Burkitt's lymphoma and cervical cancer. However, to prove that a virus causes cancer in man is quite difficult, because one cannot inoculate a disease-free human with a suspected virus, as can be done with animals. In a few cases, whereas it seems certain that particular cancers are caused by viruses, it is unlikely that viruses play a significant role in most human cancers. However, it is important to determine with assurance whether a particular type of cancer is caused by a virus, because if that is so, immunization with appropriate vaccines becomes a distinct possibility. This has been accomplished in animals: for example, whole flocks of chickens have been protected against a leukemia-like disease by using a vaccine made from certain herpes viruses.

BASIC TERMS

A few basic terms will be needed in this book for our discussion of cancer. They are defined in this section. Strictly speaking, the term tumor refers to any swollen tissue, arising from hemorrhage, inflammation, cell growth, or cancer. However, usually the term tumor refers to newly grown tissue that arises by cell division. Another term for such new growth is neoplasm. A benign neoplasm, or benign tumor, is a mass of cells that grows slowly, does not spread, and does not threaten the survival of the host. A wart is an example of a benign tumor. A malignant neoplasm, or malignant tumor, is a term equivalent to cancer; it is a mass of cells able to spread to other parts of the body and threaten the survival of the host. It need not to have begun to spread to be called cancer. Spreading can occur by two processes: invasion and metastasis. Invasion is simple expansion into surrounding tissues. Metastasis is the spread of cancer cells to distant sites not directly connected to the original cancer; it usually occurs either via blood and lymph vessels or by direct release into body cavities. The conversion of a normal cell to a tumor cell is called transformation. A tumor arising from a transformed cell at the original site of the transformation is called a primary cancer; tumors arising at distant sites as a result of metastasis are called secondary tumors.

ADDITIONAL READINGS

American Cancer Society. 1977. "Lung cancer and smoking." In Cancer Facts and Figures. New York. p. 19.

Berenblum, I. 1974. <u>Carcinogenesis as a Biological Problem</u>. North-Holland.

Burbank, F. 1971. "Patterns in cancer mortality in the United States, 1950-1967." Natl. Cancer Inst. Monograph.

<u>Cancer Facts and Figures</u>. 1980-1985. American Cancer Society.

Fraumeni, J. F. 1975. <u>Persons at High Risk of Cancer</u>. Academic Press.

Ruddon, R.W. 1981. <u>Cancer Biology</u>. Oxford Press.

2

A Review of
Cell Biology

Chapter 1 presented an introduction to several facets of cancer biology. In order to examine these features in greater depth, an understanding of cell biology is required. This chapter is designed to fill that need for the reader who either has not taken a formal course in cell biology or for whom a review of the material would be valuable. Those already having an adequate background can omit this chapter.

THE CELL THEORY

The term cell was introduced by Robert Hooke in 1665. By examining thin slices of cork and other plant tissues with a simple microscope, Hooke observed porelike or box-like units that resembled cells in a monastery or prison. The most extensive early observations were made by Antonie van Leeuwenhoek (starting in 1673 and continuing for more than 25 years), who discovered single-celled organisms in stagnant water, infusions, and scrapings from teeth. During the next century microscopes were considerably improved, enabling observations to be made that showed more detail of the structure of individual cells, such as the fact that every animal and plant cell contains a nucleus. Between 1838 and 1839, M. Schleiden and T. Schwann examined a wide variety of organisms and tissues and formalized the cell theory, which stated that all living organisms consist of cells and that cells are the basic units of the structure and function of all living tissue. Observations made by R. Virchow in 1855 led to the proposal that all cells arise from pre-existing cells. This hypothesis was confirmed by Flemming, who first observed cell division; in the 1870s, he introduced the term mitosis to describe the process in which threadlike structures (chromosomes) split lengthwise and become distributed to the two daughter cells. Between 1885 and 1905, a variety of studies of both fertilization of an egg by sperm and of the mode of production of eggs and sperm from precursor cells led to the discoveries that (1) following fertilization egg and sperm cell nuclei fuse, (2) the number of chromosomes in a fertilized egg is the same as that of other cells in the organism, and (3) the chromosome number in cells of the body is halved during the formation of sperm and egg.

In the latter part of the 19th century the concept of a genetic material, i.e., a substance containing the information of heredity, gradually developed, and it was recognized that the nucleus contained components that were passed on from generation to generation. In 1883 Roux made the specific suggestion that the chromosomes, which appeared in the nucleus early in mitosis, were the hereditary components in cells. A few years later, Weismann published a theory of heredity in which he proposed that chromatin (the nuclear material that appeared to condense and form chromosomes) was the hereditary material and that this material is passed from generation to generation by cellular mechanisms designed to insure that this material is precisely distributed to the daughter cells. With great insight he proposed that there were two classes of cells in the body: germ cells (those that form sperm and eggs) and "body" cells (now called somatic cells). The germ cells were responsible for carrying the hereditary material from one generation to the next.

In 1865 Gregor Mendel elegantly performed the first quantitative experiments in genetics in his studies of inheritance in garden peas. He concluded that specific units (genes) were responsible for the inheritance of particular characteristics in garden peas. His results were ignored for decades but were rediscovered in the early 1900s, after which evidence accumulated rapidly that genes were physically located on the chromosomes that are in the nucleus of cells.

GENETICS AND DNA

The birth of the science of the molecular basis of heredity began in 1871 when Friedrich Miescher isolated from the nuclei of pus cells a novel phosphorus-containing compound, which he called "nuclein." This observation was ignored until 1889 when nuclein was purified by Altmann; by detailed chemical analysis he determined that nuclein contained specific sugars and bases containing nitrogen and that it was an acidic substance. He gave nuclein a new name: nucleic acid. Later it was shown that there were two classes of nucleic acid: one contained the sugar ribose and the other had deoxyribose. The names ribose nucleic acid (RNA) and deoxyribose nucleic acid (DNA) were introduced. In 1924 Feulgen developed a chemical test for deoxyribose that could be carried out on cellular material and thereby showed that DNA is confined to the nucleus and that when chromosomes are visible, DNA is found only in chromosomes. This observation led to the first suggestion that DNA is associated with heredity, though most biologists believed that genes were made of protein. In 1944 DNA was demonstrated to be the genetic material of bacteria. However, this conclusion was not widely accepted until it was proved beyond any reasonable doubt that DNA is the genetic material of bacterial viruses. Finally, in 1953 Watson and Crick determined the structure of DNA and showed how DNA could both carry hereditary information and be replicated.

A DNA molecule consists of two long strands wrapped around one another, each in the form of a helix (Figure 2-1). Each strand is a chain made of alternating units of a phosphate group and a 5-carbon sugar (deoxyribose); to each deoxyribose is attached one of four different organic bases. The bases on one chain form weak bonds (called hydrogen bonds) to the bases on the other chain. The four bases in DNA are: adenine (A), thymine (T), guanine (G), and cytosine (C). Adenine on one chain can pair only with thymine on the other chain, and guanine on one chain can pair only with cytosine on the other chain (Figure 2-1); thus, one says that the strands are complementary. The sequence of bases in each strand of DNA and the specific pairing of bases between DNA strands account for the ability of DNA to serve as the genetic material.

An essential property of any genetic molecule is that it must be able to replicate, and the structure of DNA is well suited for replication. The details of the replication mechanism are quite complicated, but in principle the process is straightforward. An enzymatic system moves along the double helix, "looks at" the bases in each strand, and forms daughter strands by joining together building blocks called nucleotides, each of which consists of a base-

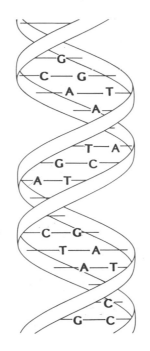

FIGURE 2-1 A diagram of a DNA molecule. The long helical strands consist of alternating sugars and phosphates.

sugar-phosphate unit. There are four DNA nucleotide building blocks, each containing one of the bases, A, T, G, and C. In order to form a faithful copy of the parental DNA molecule, the base sequence in each daughter molecule must be the same as that in the parental double helix. That is, in forming a DNA molecule nucleotides cannot be joined together by the replication machinery in a random order. In order to preserve the parental base sequence, the following occurs (Figure 2-2). As the replication enzyme reads the base sequence of the parental molecule, it selects for addition to the end of the growing strand a nucleotide that is complementary to the base in the strand being copied, according to the base-pairing rules (A pairs with T, and G pairs with C). That is, when the replication enzyme sees an AT pair in the DNA, the daughter strand copied from the parent strand with the A gets a T, and the daughter strand copied from the parental strand with the T gets an A. Thus, each parental strand serves as a template for a daughter strand with a base sequence that is complementary to that of the parental strand (actually the two daughter strands are not synthesized precisely at the same time, but this detail is unimportant for the present. In this way, each parental double-stranded molecule yields two identical daughter double-stranded molecules, and the base sequence of each daughter molecule is identical to that of the parental double helix.

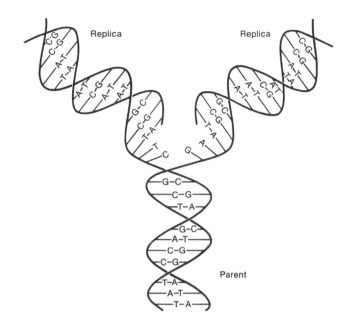

FIGURE 2-2   A diagram showing replication of a DNA molecule.

The ultimate product of almost all genes is a protein molecule. The genetic information for synthesis of each protein resides in the base sequence of DNA in that the sequence of amino acids in every protein molecule is determined by the sequence of bases in a particular segment of DNA. The relation between the base sequence in DNA and the amino acid sequence of a protein is straightforward: triplets of adjacent bases, such as CAC, TGG, AAC, etc., correspond to particular amino acids. Thus, simply by reading the bases in order, the amino acid sequence of the protein product could be determined directly. The set of all relations between base triplets and amino acids is called the genetic code. Each of the 64 possible triplets is called a codon.

For a variety of reasons, one of which is that DNA is in the nucleus and proteins are formed in the cytoplasm, the base sequence of a DNA molecule is not directly transcribed into an amino acid sequence; instead, several intermediate molecules are used. The first step in the process is the synthesis of a molecule called messenger RNA (Figure 2-3). This molecule is very similar to DNA, but with three differences: (1) It is a single-stranded molecule, also consisting of nucleotide units; (2) the sugar in RNA is ribose instead of deoxyribose; and (3) RNA does not contain the base thymine, but uses the chemically similar base uracil (U). Therefore, the bases in a messenger RNA molecule are adenine, uracil, cytosine, and guanine. Messenger RNA is synthesized in the cell nucleus in a way that is chemically similar but not identical to the mechanism of DNA synthesis.

That is, an RNA strand is copied from a template DNA molecule (just like DNA synthesis), but only one DNA strand in any given genetic segment is copied (Figure 2-4). The result is that the sequence of bases in an RNA molecule is complementary to a segment of one strand of the DNA. Base selection follows the base-pairing rules used in DNA synthesis except that uracil is substituted for thymine. That is, where there is a T in the DNA template strand, there is an A in the RNA; and an A, G, or C in DNA yields a U, C, or G, respectively, in RNA. Thus, if the sequence of bases in a DNA strand were TAATTGACG, the sequence of bases in the complementary messenger RNA strand would be AUUAACUGC. It should be noted that even though the base sequence in the messenger RNA is not the same as that in the DNA, its sequence is determined directly from the DNA and therefore it contains the same genetic information as DNA.

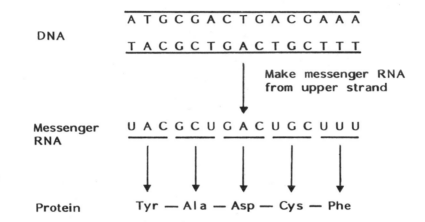

FIGURE 2-3 Synthesis of messenger RNA from DNA, and synthesis of protein from messenger RNA.

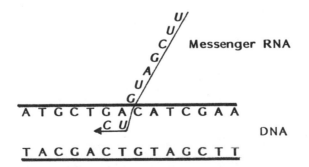

FIGURE 2-4 A messenger RNA molecule being copied from one strand of a DNA molecule. Note the complementarity of the base sequences. The arrow head shows the direction of growth of the RNA molecule.

The base sequence in a messenger RNA molecule is converted to an amino acid sequence by a complex translation system that we will examine only in outline. There are 20 amino acids found in proteins (Table 2-1), and each amino acid corresponds in the genetic code to one or more triplets of bases in RNA (Table 2-2). For example, the amino acid histidine corresponds to both CAU and CAC. Thus, an RNA molecule with the sequence AUG CCC ACU UUA UAC would cause the protein methionine-proline-threonine-leucine-tyrosine to be made.

We have seen that messenger RNA is made by direct copying of a DNA strand using base pairing to direct selection of nucleotides.

TABLE 2-1 The 20 amino acids found in proteins and their abbreviations in ().

Alanine (Ala)	Leucine (Leu)
Arginine (Arg)	Lysine (Lys)
Asparagine (Asn)	Methionine (Met)
Aspartic acid (Asp)	Phenylalanine (Phe)
Cysteine (Cys)	Proline (Pro)
Glutamic acid (Glu)	Serine (Ser)
Glutamine (Gln)	Threonine (Thr)
Glycine (Gly)	Tryptophan (Trp)
Histidine (His)	Tyrosine (Tyr)
Isoleucine (Ile)	Valine (Val)

TABLE 2-2   The genetic code

First position (5′ end)	Second position				Third position (3′ end)
	U	C	A	G	
U	Phe	Ser	Tyr	Cys	U
	Phe	Ser	Tyr	Cys	C
	Leu	Ser	Stop	Stop	A
	Leu	Ser	Stop	Trp	G
C	Leu	Pro	His	Arg	U
	Leu	Pro	His	Arg	C
	Leu	Pro	Gln	Arg	A
	Leu	Pro	Gln	Arg	G
A	Ile	Thr	Asn	Ser	U
	Ile	Thr	Asn	Ser	C
	Ile	Thr	Lys	Arg	A
	Met	Thr	Lys	Arg	G
G	Val	Ala	Asp	Gly	U
	Val	Ala	Asp	Gly	C
	Val	Ala	Glu	Gly	A
	Val	Ala	Glu	Gly	G

Note: The boxed codons are used for initiation.

Such a mechanism does not work for the synthesis of proteins, since amino acids do not interact directly with RNA. Protein synthesis is an amazingly complex process that involves more than 100 components. Suffice it to say that the messenger RNA is "read" in codon units, and each amino acid is added to the end of a growing protein chain according to the correspondences set down in Table 2-2.

MUTATION

The properties of cells are basically determined by the proteins contained in them. Many of the structural elements of cells are proteins or at least contain proteins, and almost all chemical reactions in cells are the result of the activity of specialized proteins called enzymes. A simple bacterium contains more than 1000 different enzymes. Regulatory elements comprise another category of proteins; molecules of this class determine, either directly or indirectly, whether a particular gene is active (that is, whether messenger RNA is made from the gene) and how active it is (how many RNA and protein molecules are made from the gene).

Changes in cellular proteins often change the properties of cells and may even determine whether a cell can survive. For example, if a cell lost an enzyme needed to synthesize a critical intracellular molecule, the cell would die. Sometimes, survival depends on the environment. For example, if a bacterium lost the ability to synthesize the amino acid leucine, it would be able to grow in beef soup, which is quite rich in leucine, but in other environments lacking leucine, it would be unable to grow.

We noted earlier that the amino acid sequence of a protein is determined by the base sequence of a gene. Furthermore, the properties of a protein molecule are determined almost exclusively by its sequence of amino acids. In fact, a change in the position or identity of a single amino acid can completely destroy the biological function of the protein (though it will not always do so, since some amino acid substitutions can be tolerated to some extent). Thus, it is possible for a single base change in a DNA molecule to alter cellular properties. For example, suppose the amino acid sequence of a critical portion of a protein was alanine-tryptophan-cysteine-valine and was determined by a DNA base sequence CGA ACC ACA CAA from which the RNA sequence GCU UGG UGU GUU was copied. If in the course of replicating a DNA molecule the underlined C did not appear in a daughter DNA molecule, but instead an A were present, the DNA sequence would be CGA AAC ACA CAA, the RNA sequence would be GCU UUG UGU GUU, and the amino acid sequence would be alanine-leucine-cysteine-valine. It would be quite likely that the protein would lose all of its biological activity by the substitution of leucine for tryptophan. Note that since the base sequence of the DNA has been changed in the generation of a progeny molecule, all subsequent DNA molecules derived from this daughter molecule will also contain the altered sequence and produce the altered protein. A heritable change in the properties of a cell is called a mutation; all mutations involve changes in the base sequence of DNA.

There are several possible consequences of a mutational change. One is that nothing happens at all. Since each of us has one set of chromosomes (and genes) from the mother and one set from the father, the effect of mutation in a corresponding gene in one chromosome is often nil, because the specific gene on the other chromosome is normal and allows the cell to produce enough of the normal protein to prevent any problems. A second possibility is that the cell does not survive; for example, half the normal amount of a protein may be insufficient, or the altered protein might have deleterious effects. A third possibility is that the cell survives, but its properties change. This is the consequence that will concern us in this book; that is, a mutation occurs that alters the regulation of cell division, and a normal cell begins to grow without restraint, forming a cancer.

DIFFERENTIAL GENE ACTIVITY

In the preceding question we implied that all genes are not equally active and that their activity might be regulated. This is indeed the case. This phenomenon has been studied most carefully in bacteria in which on-off activity has been observed. For example, the enzymes responsible for metabolizing the milk sugar lactose are not made by bacteria unless lactose is present. The rationale is simply not to waste energy making something that is not needed. In animal cells we can consider a more profound type of regulation by asking a simple question. If all the cells in our body are produced from a single fertilized egg and if all these cells contain the same DNA molecules (and hence the same genes), how then do cells become different? That is, why are there skin cells, nerves, stomach linings, and muscles? The process of cells becoming different during the development of an organism is called differentiation. It is explained conceptually by the observation that in no cell are all genes active and in certain cells only particular genes become activated. How this is accomplished and how it is programmed are major questions of modern biological research, and we are only beginning to get hints at the answers. What is clear, however, is that for the most part, cells differ because different messenger RNA molecules are made, and hence different proteins are present in each cell type. For example, blood cells contain the protein hemoglobin, whereas muscle cells contain the muscle protein myosin.

A variety of signals mediate the synthesis of particular messenger RNA molecules. Some of them have been identified. For example, many messenger RNA molecules are synthesized only in response to particular hormones, such as the sex hormones, which are intimately involved in the development of eggs from precursor cells and of tissues responsible for the secondary sex characteristics of adults. The hormones do not act directly on DNA in determining whether a particular messenger RNA molecules is to be synthesized; instead, regulatory proteins that either turn RNA synthesis on or off are activated or deactivated by hormones.

We will see later in this book that understanding various modes of differentiation and of regulation is probably important in combating cancer, since cancer cells have invariably not only lost many of their controls but also reacquired characteristics of embryonic cells. At the end of this chapter, embryological development will be reviewed briefly in an effort to aid the student in appreciating this apparent reversion to a more primitive state.

CELL STRUCTURE AND CELLULAR COMPONENTS

Cells are not homogeneous masses of material but have a great deal of internal structure. Since cancer cells often differ from normal cells in particular structural features, we will examine some aspects of cell structure, in particular, those of concern to cancer biology.

Cytoskeleton

A major advance in cell biology in recent years was the discovery that most mammalian cells possess a system of oriented filaments that form an internal network, called the cytoskeleton, and an elucidation of its biochemistry, organization, and function. Cytoskeletal elements include two classes of filamentous structures, microtubules and microfilaments. These structures are considerably less organized and even absent in many types of cancer cells. The significance of this difference is not well understood but will be discussed in Chapter 4.

Microtubules are cylinders about 250 angstrom units in diameter and are composed of globular subunits of a protein called tubulin. These cylinders make up cilia, flagella, and mitotic spindles. In addition, as part of the internal network of the cell, microtubules contribute in part to the shape of individual cell types; changes in their organization may be responsible for some of the changes in cell shape that occur both during embryonic development and in the everyday life of a cell.

Microfilaments are filamentous structures made of a protein called G-actin, which is also a major component of muscle fibers. They are commonly present in cells as rods 30–80 angstroms in diameter, though thicker filaments are also present. Microfilaments are linear aggregates of G-actin subunits. These subunits polymerize in certain conditions, and in other the filaments dissociate. How polymerization is regulated within cells is unknown and is an active field of research. It is considered important in cancer biology since in many types of cancer cells the G-actin subunits of microfilaments are present, but polymerization of these subunits into the microfilaments does not occur.

Cell Membrane

The outer layer of animal cells, the cell membrane, has two important functions in cell biology: it determines what molecules can enter and leave a cell, and it is the element of both cell contact and cell adhesion. It is of special interest in cancer biology, since cell adhesion is considerably weaker between cancer cells than between normal cells. As will be seen in later chapters, many of the abnormal aspects of tumor cells can be associated with alterations in the structure and function of the cell membrane and the cell surface.

Cell membranes consist primarily of molecules called lipids, which are linear molecules containing a charged end and a long fairly insoluble uncharged tail (Figure 2-5). The most elementary cell membrane consists of two layers of lipid molecules (it is usually called a lipid bilayer). The slightly charged portions of each lipid molecule are on the surface and the uncharged tails are internal. In biological membranes various proteins and glycoproteins (proteins with attached sugars) are embedded (Figure 2-6). Some of the proteins are exclusively on the membrane surface (peripheral proteins); others usually pass partly or completely through the membrane (integral proteins). The cell membrane definitely has an inside and an outside

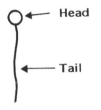

FIGURE 2-5 A schematic diagram of a lipid molecule, showing the soluble, charged, terminal "head" and the insoluble, uncharged "tail."

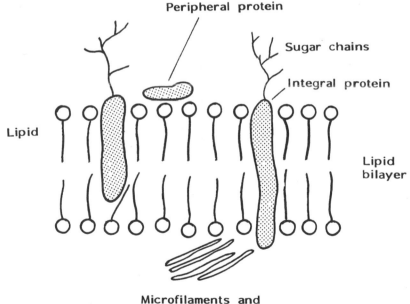

FIGURE 2-6 The structure of a biological membrane according to the fluid mosaic model.

with respect to the cell. The sugar portions of the glycoproteins are primarily on the outside, and the inside is often associated with microfilaments and microtubules. The cell membrane is a loose structure, with many fluidlike properties, in which the integral proteins and glycoproteins can move laterally in the lipid phase. This movement may be restricted by microtubules and microfilaments that may anchor some of the surface proteins from the cytoplasmic side of the membrane. The fluid nature of the membrane and the existence of mobile proteins within the membrane and on the surface was first proposed by G. Nicholson and S.J. Singer and is called the fluid mosaic model.

It is worth examining some of the experimental evidence for the fluid mosaic model, since many of these experiments, or variants thereof, were repeated in comparisons of normal and cancer cells. A particularly elegant experiment indicated that the cell surface has fluid properties. By injecting purified cell-surface proteins into rabbits L. Frye and M. Edidin prepared antibodies (a type of protein of the immune system) that specifically bind to these proteins. These antibodies were then chemically coupled to fluorescent dyes. Addition of one of these fluorescent antibodies to a sample of cells made the cells fluorescent (when viewed in a microscope able to detect fluorescence) if the cells had on their surface the protein to which the antibody had been prepared (i.e., the one administered to the rabbit). By using a variety of proteins isolated from the surfaces of different cell types, they were able to prepare fluorescent stains directed against each protein. They then made use of an interesting property of a virus called Sendai virus. When a sample of cells is infected with Sendai virus that have been killed by ultraviolet light, cells that are in contact frequently fuse. The nuclei merge, forming a single nucleus containing the chromosomes of both cells, and the cytoplasm mixes. These cells survive and are fairly stable, though some of the extra chromosomes are lost during subsequent rounds of cell division. Sendai virus will fuse cells from different species, for example, human and mouse cells. In the experiment of Frye and Edidin (Figure 2-7) mouse-human hybrid cells were formed by this fusion technique, and then fluorescent antibodies directed against either mouse or human surface proteins were applied (separately) to the fused cells. If only fluorescent antibodies directed against mouse proteins were applied, immediately after fusion, only half of the cell was fluorescent, indicating that the mouse proteins were localized in the half of the cell membrane obtained from the mouse cell. A similar result was obtained with fluorescent antibodies to human proteins; that is, only the human half of the cell was fluorescent. However, when either antibody was applied, over the next half hour the fluorescence· spread from the initially fluorescent half of the cell over the entire cell; this observation meant that both mouse and human surface proteins were capable of free motion through the membrane until they were intimately mixed. This could only occur if the lipid molecules of the membrane were so loosely bound to one another that the membrane was like a liquid. An interesting quantitative measurement was possible in this experiment: namely, from the rate of intermixing of the surface proteins it was possible to estimate how

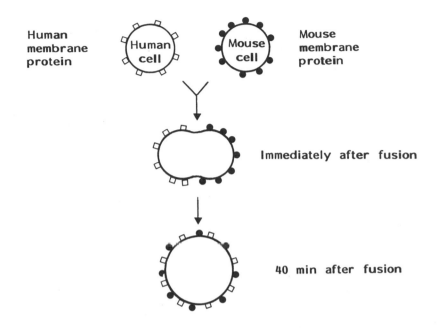

FIGURE 2-7 Drifting of surface proteins following fusion of a human and mouse cells.

freely the molecules move. Careful analysis of this and other experiments carried out under a variety of conditions has indicated that all parts of the surface are not equally fluid and that certain surface proteins are anchored by cytoskeletal elements that appear to restrict their movement.

It was pointed out above that some of the proteins and lipids of the cell surface have sugar chains attached. These sugar chains and especially the terminal sugars of the chains may be responsible for at least some features of cell adhesion. Some of the molecular models that have been proposed to explain adhesion of cells in embryos and tumors, as will be seen, place a great deal of importance on the role of the surface sugars in adhesion mechanisms.

Lysosomes

Lysosomes are membrane-bounded sacs within the cell that contain degradative enzymes. Typical enzymes contained in the lysosomes are those that digest proteins, polysaccharides, lipids, phosphate esters, and nucleic acids. These sacs serve to break down debris, fragments of cellular organelles, microorganisms, and other material that may need to be removed from the cytoplasm. When such materials contact the cell surface, often tiny regions of the cell membrane fold inward, surrounding the substances and bringing them into the cell. These membrane-bounded sacs then fuse with lysosomes, digestion of the material proceeds by the action of the lysosomal enzymes, the lysosome then fuses with the cell membrane, and the digested waste is extruded from the cell. White blood cells have particularly active lysosomes; these cells fight infection and disease by engulfing bacteria and digesting them.

Some cells are scheduled to die in the normal course of development. For example, the tail of a tadpole self-destructs as the tadpole becomes a frog. Regions of bone also die at certain times, as do specific embryonic structures that are no longer needed. In all of these cases of programmed cell death, lysosomal enzymes appear to participate in the breakdown of the cells.

Many types of cancer cells possess and excrete increased amounts of proteases (enzymes that degrade proteins). Possibly these cells may possess either abnormal lysosomes or excessive quantities of these structures. Increased levels of surface proteases may play a key role in the invasive behavior of cancer cells, so lysosomes may be one of the keys to the altered behavior of cancer cells.

THE CELL CYCLE

The biochemical events that are important for cell growth and duplication do not occur at random times. The sequence of events is called the cell cycle. Cancer cells and normal cells show significant differences in certain portions of the cell cycle. For this reason, a large research effort is devoted to understanding the controls of the cycling.

The life cycle of multiplying cells of higher organisms can be thought of as having two phases: interphase, in which most of the growth occurs, and mitosis, in which chromosomes separate and cells divide. The interphase period is 20-50 hours and mitosis takes a few hours, the particular lengths depending on the cell type. Prior to mitosis, DNA duplication must occur. However, DNA synthesis does not occur immediately before mitosis but near the middle of the interphase period (Figure 2-8). The stage of the cell cycle in which DNA replicates is designated S. Prior to the S phase is a period termed G_1 (gap 1) in which many biochemical events occur including those necessary for starting DNA synthesis. The period following DNA synthesis and mitosis is called G_2 (gap 2); this is also an active period of biosynthesis, during which, among other things, the cell prepares for mitosis. Although many things occur during the cell cycle, if one considers only DNA synthesis and cell division, the cycle consists of, in order, preparation for DNA replication (G_1), replication (S), preparation for mitosis (G_2), mitosis (M), and cell division (D), after which the cell enters the G_1 phase again.

Except for certain cells in the adult body, (for example, those that form blood cells or regenerate the lining of the intestine, and liver cells), most differentiated cells rarely duplicate their DNA or divide. This stationary state of the cell is reached after cell division and in the G_1 stage. Stationary cells are considered to have left the cell cycle and to have entered a phase of specialized function called G_0 (Figure 2-8). Neither the biochemical events that regulate the normal cell cycle nor the nature of the transition to G_0 are known. Clearly, this knowledge is essential to understanding cancer, especially

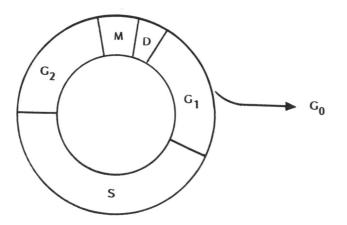

FIGURE 2-8 The cell cycle.

since transformation of normal cells to cancer cells probably involves a departure from G_0 and reentry into G_1. In a later section we will also see that cancer cells often move from M to S with a G_1 phase that is much shorter than that of those cells that are still dividing in the adult. Presumably, biochemical events that regulate DNA synthesis in normal cells during G_1 are aberrant in cancer cells.

EMBRYONIC DEVELOPMENT

In Chapter 4 we will see that cancer cells show certain features in common with embryonic cells. Understanding both this phenomenon and the proposed mechanisms by which specific cancers are derived from particular tissues will be facilitated by a summary of the phases of early embryonic development.

The embryo begins life as a fertilized egg produced by the union of egg and sperm. The fertilized egg next undergoes a period of rapid division in which the cell number in the embryo increases without any significant increase in the total amount of material present. This period is termed cleavage, and the result is a solid ball of cells. Internal movement of the cells results in the formation of a hollow cavity (Figure 2-9). The hollow ball is called a blastula. At this point, major rearrangements of the location of cells occurs, and the embryo begins to change in form. The first result is a cuplike structure (the gastrula), which then continues to fold until the cup closes. Note that this structure (late gastrula) is layered in the sense that the cells have three distinct locations and origins: outer cells, which arose from the outside of the cup; the innermost cells, which arose from the inside of the cup and line the cavity of the late gastrula; and middle cells, which consist of all of the inner cells of the blastula. These three layers are collectively called germ layers and are individually the ectoderm (outside), mesoderm (middle), and endoderm (inside). As the embryo continues to develop, each of these layers forms tissues of specific types; that is, their destiny is already

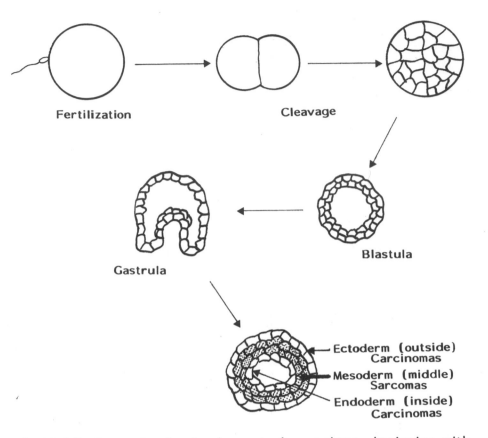

FIGURE 2-9 Stages in the development of an embryo, beginning with fertilization.

programmed at this stage. The ectoderm gives rise to three classes of tissue: the nervous system, a group of cells called the neural crest (which forms some nerve cells, pigment cells, and some connective tissue), and the outer skin and its derivatives. The endoderm develops into the gut tube and all of its derivatives. The mesoderm produces the major structures and organs, such as the inner part of the skin (dermis), muscles, skeleton, heart, blood vessels, kidneys, and gonads. Such tissue differentiation occurs because only certain genes in cells in the different parts of the embryo become activated. This activation leads to the synthesis of the particular proteins that make cells specialized and different. In this way cells with the same set of genes can become different.

Cancer cells are usually classified according to the embryonic tissue of origin. That is, carcinomas are cancers of tissues derived from ectoderm and endoderm, and sarcomas are cancers of tissue derived from mesoderm. This classification is based in part on the fact that reactivation of genes that were only active in the embryo may be a cause of some cancers, as will be seen in later chapters.

ADDITIONAL READINGS

Alberts, B., D. Bray, J. Lewis, M. Raff, K. Roberts, and J.D. Watson. 1983. Molecular Biology of the Cell. Garland.

Dyson, R.D. 1978. Cell Biology: A Molecular Approach. Allyn and Bacon.

Freifelder, D. 1985. Essentials of Molecular Biology. Jones and Bartlett.

Oppenheimer, S.B. and G. Lefevre. 1980. Introduction to Embryonic Development. Allyn and Bacon.

3

Theories of the Cause of Cancer

Numerous hypotheses have been advanced to explain cancer in biochemical terms. We will not consider all of them in this chapter but instead group the ideas into two major models for the cause of cancer. The first is that certain alterations of the genetic material can cause cancer. These alterations include the addition of new genetic material (such as viral genes), deletion of genes, and changing genes by point mutations or chromosomal rearrangements (Figure 3-1). The second model is that normal genes are either activated or repressed, without alteration of DNA structure. In both classes of models the events must lead to breakdown of growth control in the cells, so that cells with malignant behavior result.

We begin with considering some of the evidence for the two models. In thinking about the models one must keep in mind that both classes of models may provide explanations for particular cancers, since a great deal of evidence suggests that there are many pathways by which a normal cell can become cancerous and that cancer cells are extraordinarily variable. The minimal requirement is only that a defect must occur in the mechanism by which cell growth is controlled.

THE THEORY OF GENE ALTERATION

A large body of evidence supports the idea that alterations of genetic material can cause cancer. Before the discovery of oncogenes, which will be described in Chapter 8, most of the evidence was indirect or correlative, though taken in its entirety the evidence has always been substantial. An important point that pervades this way of thinking is that most malignant transformation is stable and inherited by progeny cells, just as genetic alterations are invariably stable.

Normal chromosome

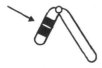

Point change

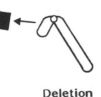

Deletion

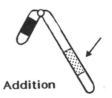

Addition

FIGURE 3-1 Three of several known types of changes that occur in the chromosomes of cells that have become cancerous.

Four general classes of evidence support the notion that an alteration in the genetic material can cause cancer. These include:

1. Cancer is induced by radiation that damages DNA.
2. Cancer is induced by chemicals that damage DNA.
3. Cancer is induced by addition of DNA to cells.
4. Some cancers are inherited as a single gene.

At this point in the book we will examine some of the key findings that support these statements. In Chapters 6-8 we will expand on these topics. Here we are mainly concerned with understanding the basis for the initial event that converts a normal cell to the cancerous state. Because the alteration is thought of as a transformation, it is common to refer to a cancer cell as a transformed cell and to the process as transformation. The terms malignant transformation and neoplastic ("new tissue") transformation are equivalent and common medical terms.

Thousands of carcinogenic (cancer-causing) chemicals are known. Studies of the interaction of many of these with purified DNA and examination of the DNA of cells treated with the chemicals have shown that many carcinogens damage DNA. Furthermore, the effectiveness of the carcinogen is often directly correlated with its ability to interact with and damage DNA. For example, several carcinogens react strongly with the guanine in DNA and thereby alter the DNA. Radiation such as ultraviolet light and x rays are also carcinogenic. Irradiation of both free DNA and of living cells causes damage to the DNA. Cells contain mechanisms for repairing most radiation-damaged DNA, and failure to enact repair often increases the frequency of cancer. For example, patients with the disease xeroderma pigmentosum are unable to repair damage from ultraviolet light and have a very high incidence of radiation-induced skin cancer. In bacteria, repair of badly damaged DNA often occurs by what is known as an error-prone repair mechanism; the structural integrity of the DNA is not restored, but replication is allowed to proceed past damage that ordinarily stops replication, with occasional insertion of incorrect bases in daughter DNA molecules. Thus, mutations result. This mode of repair has not yet been detected in human cells but may be important in radiation-induced mutagenesis and in cell transformation. Radiation can also activate viruses present in the cells of some strains of animals and cause leukemia (for example, in cats and mice). Additional evidence for the relation between cancer and radiation damage to DNA is that the wavelengths of ultraviolet light that are effective in inducing skin tumors in mice are the same wavelengths that are absorbed by and damage DNA.

The cells of many organisms that have been transformed to the cancerous state by chemicals, radiation, and virus infection often show distinct chromosomal abnormalities, such as chromosome breaks, exchange of fragments between chromosomes, and extra chromosomes, again supporting the idea that the genetic material is indeed altered by cancer-inducing agents (Figure 3-1).

Chromosomal abnormalities are observed in many cancer cells (Figure 3-2), and in fact the existence of these abnormalities is often

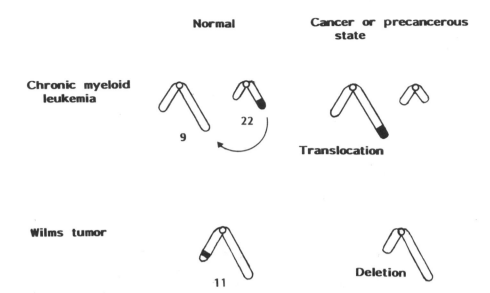

Normal

Cancer or precancerous state

Chronic myeloid leukemia

9

22

Translocation

Wilms tumor

11

Deletion

FIGURE 3-2 Chromosome abnormalities in two different human cancers. In cancer cells of patients with chronic myeloid leukemia the end of the long arm of chromosome 22 has been translocated to the end of the long arm of chromosome 9. In cell with people with Wilms' tumor a portion of chromosome 11 is missing.

used in cancer diagnosis. For example, in chronic myeloid leukemia, a significant number of patients have the long arm of chromosome 22 shortened as the result of a piece of this arm being moved to the end of the long arm of chromosome 9. It has also been observed that individuals who have this chromosomal abnormality, but are free of the leukemia, almost always develop the disease at a later time. In addition to this abnormality in chromosome 22, patients with certain forms of leukemia have an extra chromosome 8 (three copies instead of two) and an altered chromosome 17. Patients with meningioma usually lack a portion of either chromosome 22 or chromosome 8, and patients with Burkitt's lymphoma usually have an altered chromosome 14. Unfortunately, lack of these abnormalities does not mean that a person is free of these cancers, since numerous patients with the specific cancers mentioned have none of the chromosomal abnormalities just described. Recent studies have indicated that associated with exchanges of chromosomal segments and chromosome breakage is an adjacent piece of DNA called an oncogene. These elements will be described in Chapter 8. Cells from elderly people usually have more chromosomal abnormalities than those from the young; this observation may be related to the fact that older individuals are at greatly increased risk of developing many cancers.

Cancer is also associated with increased numbers of chromosomes. For example, there is a greater incidence of leukemia in patients with three copies of certain chromosomes (such as the extra chromosome

21 that is responsible for Down syndrome) rather than the normal two. An extensive study of hundreds of cancer patients has shown that almost all cancer cells examined have more chromosomes than normal cells (the cells are said to be aneuploid). The significance of the greater number of chromosomes is unclear, but several suggestions have been made: (1) alterations in chromosomes or chromosome numbers may directly induce cancer, (2) alterations may predispose the individual to other agents that induce the cancer, (3) chromosomal alterations might confer a selective growth advantage on a partially transformed cell, and (4) cancer cells might make frequent errors in mitosis, resulting in accumulation of extra chromosomes. A significant observation is that many human cancers do not exhibit consistent chromosomal abnormalities. This has been taken to mean that there are many different alterations of genetic information that can interfere with the control of cell growth. In Chapter 8, where oncogenes are discussed, we will see that this is indeed the case.

Some cancers usually progress from a state of lower malignancy to a more rapidly growing, more malignant state. This can be seen by removing tumor cells and transplanting them several times through different animals. In one experiment, early sarcomas in mice were removed, a piece of tissue of known size was transplanted to another mouse, and the time required to grow to a particular size was measured. The new tumor was then excised, a portion was transplanted to another mouse, and again the growth rate was measured. This transplant procedure was repeated several times, each time using a new mouse, and it was found that later transplants grew successively more rapidly and were more malignant (spread more) than the earlier transplants. Examination of the chromosomes of the tumor cells in various transplants showed that cells in the later transplants had more extra chromosomes and more abnormal chromosomes. Such evidence indirectly suggests that increased malignancy may be related to changes in the genetic material. Note that for two reasons this sort of finding does not prove that the altered chromosomes are the cause of the malignant state: (1) in the early transplants chromosome abnormalities may have been present but not grossly visible and (2) the increase in growth rate may have been the cause of, rather than caused by, the abnormalities.

Several examples of mutations that are always associated with cancer also support the gene alteration hypothesis. In the fruit fly, a specific type of cancer of cells that develop into the brain occurs in about 25 percent of all the offspring of a male and female fly that each carry a specific single mutated gene. In these cases, the future brain cells divide in an uncontrolled manner and kill the larva before it reaches adulthood. Genetic experiments indicate that the single mutation arises in a gene that is normally required to control the growth of the brain cells.

In humans, a specific cancer of the eye called bilateral retinoblastoma is associated with presence of a particular mutation. A disease called familial polyposis, in which large numbers of polyps form in the large intestine and rectum is also a result of the presence of a particular altered gene. Whereas these polyps are not cancers, failure to remove them before the age of 40 results in nearly 100 percent of the patients developing cancer of the bowel. There is also a predisposition in these patients to develop cancer of the skin and bone. Other examples will be described in Chapter 7.

A well-studied cancer that suggests that alteration of genetic material is a primary causative factor is melanoma in the platy, a tropical fish. Melanoma, a cancer of pigment cells of the skin, does not occur frequently in the platy. Another fish, the swordtail, can be mated with the platy and will produce viable offspring. These hybrid offspring have rapidly dividing pigment cells in the dorsal fin area. If such a hybrid platy is once again crossed with a swordtail, the pigment cells in the dorsal fin area divide so extensively that tumors are formed in many of these hybrids, killing the fish. A likely explanation for these results (but not the only explanation) is that the platy seldom gets melanoma because it possesses regulatory genes that control proliferation of pigment cells. The swordtail does not have pigment cells in the dorsal fin area and thus never evolved to possess these regulatory genes. Hybrids resulting from crosses between a platy and a swordtail have pigment cells, but also a reduced number of the regulatory genes. Continued crossing of the hybrid platy with a swordtail further dilutes the regulatory genes, leading to a failure in the control of pigment cell proliferation, that is, development of cancer.

In summary, each piece of evidence presented in this section is indirect and, by itself, inconclusive. However, taken as a whole, a good case can be made for the conclusion that many cancers may be, at least in part, caused by an alteration of the genetic material in cells. It may be that alteration of genetic material is the initial step in some forms of carcinogenesis and that other factors are required to promote the formation of a clinically defined cancer. In Chapters 6 and 8 we will examine such "two-step" processes that appear to be involved in the formation of some cancers.

THE GENE ACTIVATION THEORY

In higher organisms all cells are derived from the fertilized egg by repeated cycles of DNA replication and mitosis, which provides all daughter cells with identical sets of DNA. Thus, all cells in an organism contain the same genes (except for sperm and egg, which have only a single set of chromosomes), so it is reasonable to ask why individual cells are of such different types. That is, how do muscle cells, nerve cells, and blood cells all develop from a population of cells containing identical base sequences in their DNA? In principle, the answer to this question of cell differentiation is simple: only certain genes in certain cells become activated, whereas others are repressed. In this way a particular type of cell can synthesize the specific proteins needed for its specialized function. More detailed information is unfortunately not available.

The same mechanisms of differential gene activation and repression that direct cells in the embryo to become different may also be involved in the development of some cancers. The idea is that some proteins not present in normal cells are present in cancer cells and that some proteins present in normal cells are absent in cancer cells. This hypothesis, the gene activation theory, is shown schematically in Figure 3-3. The essential feature of the hypothesis is that only the expression of genes, rather than the genetic material itself, is altered.

What is the evidence that supports the gene activation model? Major support comes from analysis of the proteins (in particular, surface proteins) made by some cancer cells and by the normal cells from which they are derived: some normal proteins are not present and some proteins found only in normal embryonic cells are present, as proposed in Figure 3-3. Of course, one cannot conclude that the production of the embryonic proteins and the loss of normal proteins is the cause of transformation; rather, it could be the result of the conversion.

Other significant observations are those concerned with the reversibility of the cancerous state. The reasoning is that if a group of cancer cells could easily revert to normal cells under specific growth conditions, the genetic material in these cells could not have been altered. Transformation to the cancerous state by activation of specific genes and repression of others is consistent with observations of reversibility. That is, by deactivation of cancer genes in cancer cells and reactivation of the normal genes, a cancer cell could be converted to a normal cell. Before presenting some of the observations of reversibility, we must stress that even though gene activation and

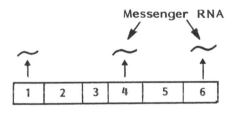

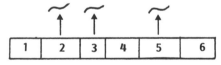

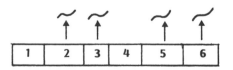

FIGURE 3-3 A gene activation model of cancer. Genes active in embryonic cells (gene 6) and no longer expressed in adult cells are turned on, causing conversion of a normal cell to a cancer cell.

repression may be involved in some cancers and may even be the
cause of selected cancers, it is unlikely that gene activation can
account for the development of many cancers because of the substantial
evidence that supports the gene alteration model.

The main evidence for reversion of cancer cells to the normal
comes from studies of one specific tumor, the mouse teratoma
(teratocarcinoma), a rather unusual type of tumor. Teratomas are
tumors derived from germ cells. These tumors often are
indistinguishable from early embryos and may in fact develop rather
normally like embryos if they are maintained in the proper place in
the body. Teratomas and other tumors also often resemble embryos
in terms of the presence of specific cell surface molecules, called
embryonic antigens. (The term antigen means a molecule that can
cause production of antibodies. It is used here because these surface
molecules are usually detected by immunological tests.) Thus, some
of the same genes active in embryos are also active in tumors. Normal
adult cells seldom display these antigens. Mouse teratomas can be
isolated from the testis of some strains of young mice and can be
transplanted to other mice or maintained in culture. When teratoma
cells are inoculated into the body cavity of mice, they develop into
numerous clusters called "embryoid bodies." These free-floating
clusters resemble normal 6-day-old mouse embryos. Embryoid bodies
will begin development like normal embryos and differentiate into many
tissues if grown in the eye cavity of mice. However, if maintained in
the body cavity, embryoid bodies continue to proliferate rapidly.

K. Illmensee and B. Mintz isolated teratoma cells and injected these
cells into early mouse embryo blastocysts (a developmental stage) from
another strain of mouse. These blastocysts containing the teratoma
cells were then implanted into the uterus of other female mice. The
embryos developed into normal tumor-free adult mice. To be sure that
the teratoma cells did not simply die, genetic markers that identified
the parent animals were introduced in the experiment. The teratoma
cells were derived from mice that carried genes for specific pigments
in their fur and specific types of hemoglobin molecules. The
blastocysts were obtained from animals with white fur and a different
type of hemoglobin. The result of the experiment is shown in Figure
3-4: the mice that were born had both black and white fur and had
both types of hemoglobins, which indicated that some of their tissues
were derived from the normal mouse embryo cells and others were
derived from the teratoma cells. The mice were free of tumors, so
normal mice developed with some of their cells originating from a type
of tumor. A significant feature of this experiment is that teratoma
tumor cells differentiated into normal adult tissues, but if left in the
original place, the original teratoma cells formed a tumor. Thus, the
fate of these cells seems to depend on environmental factors. Another
experiment, this time with normal cells, supports the notion of a role
of environment. Normal 6-day-old mouse embryo cells were implanted
into the testis of an adult mouse, and these developed into a teratoma.
However, older embryo cells did not form tumors under these
conditions, so cell age is clearly also important. These experiments
indicate that young embryo cells and certain tumor cells share certain
potential and can either grow in an unregulated way or differentiate

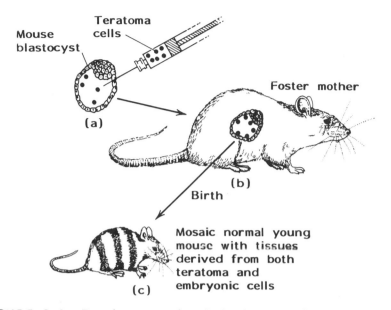

FIGURE 3-4 Development of a hybrid mouse from a mouse embryo into which teratoma cells have been injected. (a) Teratoma cells (black) are injected into a normal mouse embryo blastocyst. The teratoma cells carry a gene for dark fur, and the cells in the blastocyst carry a gene for white fur. (b) The injected embryo is grown in the uterus of a female mouse. (c) The mouse developing from the injected blastocyst lacks tumors, yet it contains tissues derived from both the teratoma cells (black fur) and from normal cells (white fur). (From Oppenheimer. 1980. <u>Introduction to Embryonic Development</u>. Allyn and Bacon.)

into normal adult tissue, depending upon the environment in which the cells reside.

Teratomas are being used in many studies designed to investigate the nature of the malignant (spreading tumor) versus the benign (nonspreading tumor) state and the conditions required for cell growth and differentiation. Teratoma cells provide excellent material for these studies, because they can be obtained in enormous numbers by growing them in the body cavity of mice or in growth medium. These cells can retain the malignant potential if maintained in the free-floating form in the body cavity or can differentiate into normal tissues if implanted into embryonic blastocysts or under the skin. For these reasons, it is likely that teratomas will provide us with many answers to the relationship between the malignant and benign state or between cell growth and cell differentiation.

These experiments suggest that in teratomas, at least, it is unlikely that irreversible genetic alterations have occurred and that teratomas probably result from activation and repression of genes by environmental factors, rather than from mutation or genetic alteration.

A few other cancers might also be caused by gene activation or repression. One is a virus-induced cancer called Lucké adenocarcinoma, which occurs quite commonly in frogs. The experimental evidence is the following. A nucleus from a Lucké adenocarcinoma cell was transplanted into a fertilized frog egg whose nucleus had been removed after fertilization (Figure 3-5). The egg with the cancer cell nucleus developed into a tadpole with no evidence of cancer in any of its tissues, so an irreversible genetic alteration did not exist in the nucleus of these cancer cells. Even in a virus-induced cancer, in which case a genetic change seems inevitable, a true genetic alteration need not always occur.

Neuroblastoma is a malignant human cancer of infants in which immature nerve cells (neuroblasts) spread rapidly throughout the body, usually causing rapid death. In some documented cases, these malignant neuroblasts spontaneously have reverted to normal nerve cells, and the child has survived. When these cells are grown in culture medium, a variety of substances cause the cancer cells to differentiate into what appear to be normal nerve cells that display no malignant characteristics. One of these substances, dimethylsulfoxide, also causes cells of a red blood cell leukemia (erythroleukemia) to differentiate into nonmalignant cells. Another substance, called MGI protein, can cause human acute myelogenous leukemia cells to differentiate into white blood cells that behave normally.

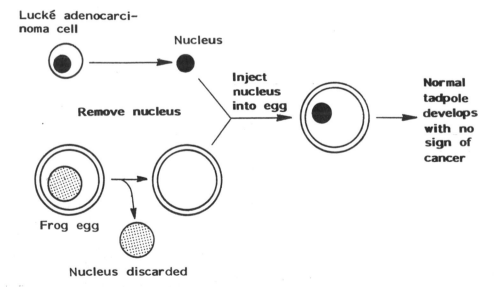

FIGURE 3-5 An experiment in support of the gene activation theory, showing that the presence of the nucleus of a cancer cell is insufficient to cause cancer. The nucleus is transplanted from a cancer cell to a fertilized egg, whose nucleus has been removed after fertilization, and a cancer-free tadpole develops.

Observations of reversibility of the transformed state do not eliminate the possibility that the origin and stable expression of the transformed state involve mutations. For example, under certain conditions, a mutation able to transform a normal cell might be actively expressed, while under other conditions it may not. Realization of the many possibilities illustrates how difficult it is to draw unambiguous conclusions about the causes of cancer.

Tumors are not confined to animal cells, for many plants also can develop tumors. These have only recently been studied in any detail. Some experiments demonstrate that plant tumor cells can also revert to normal cells, and in certain instances a single plant tumor cell can give rise to an entirely normal plant that flowers and produces normal seeds.

In some cancers, and in fact those for which reversion to normalcy has never been demonstrated, it is clear that embryonic genes are turned on. For example, liver cancer cells often possess a surface antigen identical to an antigen found on embryonic liver cells, but not on normal adult liver cells (Figure 3-6). Such findings clearly show that normal embryo genes that are repressed during adult life are reactivated in some cancers. Whether activation of these genes is a cause of the cancer, again, has not been proven. However, once one accepts the fact that some embryonic genes are reactivated, it is not unreasonable to hypothesize that other embryonic genes, such as

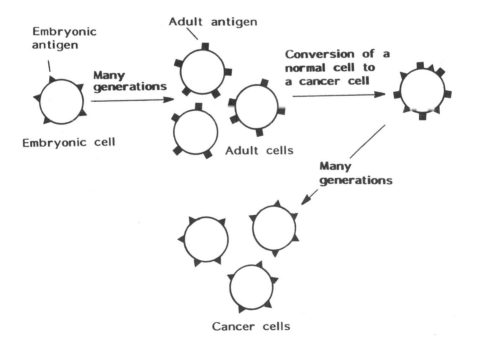

FIGURE 3-6 Embryonic surface antigens often appear on the surface of cancer cells, frequently substituting for antigens present on normal adult cells.

those needed for continuous division and cellular migration, both
properties of early embryonic cells, may also be reactivated. This
notion will be explored in later chapters.

SUMMARY

Gene alteration is a major feature of cancer induction, but gene
activation seems to be significant also, at least in some cancers. If
a cancer-inducing genetic alteration does occur, such an alteration
might not cause the cancer unless the altered gene is also activated.
Specific substances may be required to activate the altered genes and
promote development of an actual cancer. Some cancers may involve
activation of genes that are normally turned off in differentiated adult
tissues but active in embryos. It seems likely that different cancers
are caused by a variety of factors, the main requirement being
production of a defect in growth control.

ADDITIONAL READINGS

German, J. 1974. Chromosomes and Cancer. Wiley.

Hiatt, H.H., J.D. Watson, and J.A. Winsten. 1977. Origins of Human
Cancer. Cold Spring Harbor.

Martin, G.R. 1980. "Teratocarcinoma and mammalian embryogenesis."
Science, 209, 768.

Ruddon, R.W. 1981. Cancer Biology. Oxford.

Snyder, L.A., D. Freifelder, and D.L. Hartl. 1985. General Genetics.
Chapter 6. Jones and Bartlett.

4

Alterations Associated with Some Transformed Cells

Cancer cells differ from normal cells in a variety of ways. If cancer is to be understood, it is important to note these differences and to determine which properties of cancer cells are responsible for the uncontrolled growth of these cells and their dispersal through the body. This information is not yet available, so in this chapter we must be content just to look at differences between normal cells and cancer cells. To make such a comparison one would ideally want to study cells just isolated from a tumor. However, to obtain interpretable results from experiments with cells obtained directly from tissue has been exceedingly difficult, because both normal and cancerous tissue are mixtures of different types of cells; the problem is that when comparing either the biochemistry or growth characteristics of normal and cancerous tissue, one cannot be sure which cells contribute to the observed changes. Therefore, the usual approach to identifying biochemical differences between normal cells and cancer cells has been and remains to study cells grown in the laboratory in a liquid growth medium (such cells are said to be in culture), because in these cultures all cells are progeny of a single cell and hence are fairly uniform. Furthermore, in culture the environment of the cells can be both defined and experimentally manipulated (for example, a carcinogen can be added to a culture of normal cells), so it becomes possible to study the process by which a normal cell is transformed to a cancer cell.

When studying transformation in culture, some criterion is needed for determining whether conversion has occurred. A variety of tests are used, but the ultimate one is whether the cells can form a tumor when injected into a susceptible animal. Unfortunately, the relation between the observed properties of cells classified as transformed and the ability of these cells to cause a tumor is not a straightforward one. Treatment of normal cells with known carcinogens causes changes in the growth characteristics of these cells in culture that one would expect of a cancer cell, and indeed the altered cells will cause tumors when injected into an animal. However, the transformed cells invariably acquire several characteristic properties simultaneously, yet these properties are not all required for tumor formation. For example, cells transformed by a particular carcinogen may always gain characteristics A, B, C, D, and E and may cause tumors; however, from these transformed cultures one can usually select cells that have lost some of these properties (for example, having only the properties A, C, and D), yet still cause tumors to form when injected into an animal. Thus, one has the paradox that all five traits always appear together as a result of exposure to the carcinogen, but all are not necessary for tumor formation. This type of observation is one of many that has made the identification of the critical events in transformation quite difficult. In addition to this experimental complication, studies on cell cultures derived from tumors (and which retain the ability to form tumors in animals) indicate that the biochemical properties, structure, and growth habit of these cancer cell lines are quite variable from one culture to the next. The reader should not be depressed by all these precautions. As will be seen, a few characteristics, such as uncontrolled growth and immortality, are observed in all cancer cells.

DIFFERENCES IN THE GROWTH OF NORMAL AND CANCER CELLS IN CULTURE

In an animal the primary feature of a cancer cell is its uncontrolled growth, in contrast with the carefully regulated growth of normal cells. In adults (except in the case of injury), the number of new cells formed in tissues equals the number lost by cell death or exfoliation (loss of cells from surfaces). However, in cancers, cells continue to divide, not necessarily at a greater rate than normal cells but continuously and in a less regulated manner. Furthermore, the cancer cells do not acquire the structural organization of the surrounding tissue; for all practical purposes, the cells follow their own rules and form tumors that grow in size and become, as a result of their mass and eventual spread, damaging to the normal functioning of the surrounding tissues.

In this section we first examine several properties of the growth of cancer cells in culture that mimic the unregulated growth in the animal. Primary among these are (1) the so-called immortality of cancer cells, (2) the fact that, unlike normal cells, cell contact does not act as an apparent signal to stop dividing, and (3) the ability of a cancer cell to multiply without being in contact with a surface. We will then consider a variety of biochemical differences between normal and cancer cells that may be connected in some way with the growth habits of these cells. The questions that we hope to answer regard the identity of the biochemical factors that control cell division, how these factors work, and whether cancer cells lack the signals or instead lack the ability to respond to the signals.

Immortality of Transformed Cells in Culture

If one begins a culture with cells taken from embryonic tissue, most normal mammalian cells have a limited life expectancy in culture, typically 50-60 generations. After this number of generations the cells in the culture begin to die and disintegrate. Once this cell death begins, over a period of several days or weeks all cells in the culture die. The mechanism of this programmed cell death, which is called senescence, is unknown. (It is unlikely that this has anything to do with normal human mortality in that the time scale of birth to death of a human cell culture is 1-2 months.) Cells obtained from cancerous tissue do not exhibit this limited division and are considered to be immortal. Some cell cultures obtained from human and mouse cancers have been grown continually for more than 25 years, which represents nearly 10,000 generations of growth. If a large number of cultures of normal cells is examined, one usually finds that after apparent death of the cultures, one or possibly a few cells in some of the cultures survive and continue to multiply. With increasing numbers of generations stable cultures can be developed from these new cells. Notably, as the number of cells increases, the number of chromosomes per cell also increases, suggesting that a greater number of certain growth-promoting genes may be generated and selected for during continual growth of the culture. The cultures ultimately derived from these few surviving cells have two significant properties: (1) they are immortal in the sense that cell division can occur indefinitely, like cells isolated from cancerous tissue (that is, the cultures no longer exhibit senescence), and (2) if cells are injected into a large number of susceptible animals, a few percent of the animals will develop tumors. Such cultures are said to have been partially transformed; they also possess other features of transformed cells that will be described in the few sections that follow.

If a culture of normal cells is treated with a carcinogen (which may be a chemical carcinogen, radiation, or a tumor virus), over a period of about 5-14 days the culture also acquires the transformed characteristics, namely, immortality and tumor production. These observations provide the basis for confidence in studying the transformation process in culture as a means of learning about the conversion of normal cells to cancer cells.

Decreased Density-Dependent Inhibition of Growth ("Contact Inhibition")

If normal cells are placed in a glass or plastic dish containing liquid growth medium, the cells fall to the bottom of the vessel and adsorb to the surface, spreading out as they adsorb, and within 24-48 hours they begin to divide. Division continues until the cells are in contact with neighboring cells on all sides, and a layer of cells, one cell thick, called a monolayer results. Once no more space on the surface is available, cell division stops. When this phenomenon was first observed, it was thought that cell contact was the signal for turning off cell division, and the phenomenon was called contact inhibition, a term that is still commonly encountered (see below). The inhibition of division in a monolayer is no more permanent than in tissue: for example, if the monolayer is cut with a knife, damaged cells along the cut disintegrate, and cell division begins again along the cut, filling in the space. That is, "healing" occurs in the culture. The response to contact is different with cancer cells.

If cancer cells (either those obtained from a tumor or cells transformed in culture by carcinogens) are placed in a culture vessel, the initial stages of development of the monolayer are the same as with normal cells. However, when the cells come in contact, division does not stop. Instead the cells continue to divide and pile up on one another, forming a jumbled multilayer of cells that lacks any obvious organization (Figures 4-1, 4-2). Growth and division are only limited by the availability of nutrients in the medium. Contact inhibition and the lack thereof in cancer cells mimic the properties of normal and cancer cells in the body; that is, most normal cells multiply only when contact is broken by an injury, or if they are on a surface, and cancer cells grow while totally surrounded by normal tissue.

Recent experiments indicate that mere contact is not the significant factor, and the term contact inhibition is gradually being replaced by another term, density-dependent growth. All cells require nutrients, oxygen, and various growth factors for multiplication. Cells in contact with one another have less contact with the surrounding medium, and hence may be starved for essential substances simply by crowding. Cancer cells require lower concentrations of many necessary

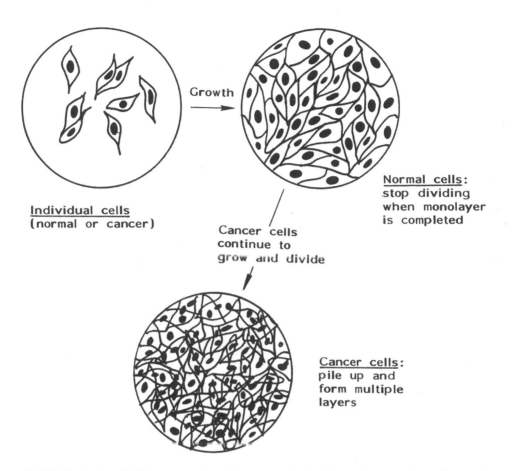

Growth

Individual cells
(normal or cancer)

Cancer cells
continue to
grow and divide

Normal cells:
stop dividing
when monolayer
is completed

Cancer cells:
pile up and
form multiple
layers

FIGURE 4-1   Differences in the growth habits of normal cells and cancer cells. Cells are shown growing on the bottom of a flat dish. The drawing is not to scale, for the cells are about 1000 times too large.

substances (as will be seen later in this chapter), so their growth may be less affected by contact than normal cells. Thus, the term density-dependent growth is considered to be a more acceptable term than contact inhibition.

Cancer cells are also held less firmly to adjacent cells than are normal cells; time-lapse photography shows that both normal and cancer cells move continually over one another. The frequency of movement is much greater in the cancer cells, which adhere to one another less tightly than normal cells (this will be discussed shortly); thus, in crowded conditions cancer cells may spend a fairly large fraction of time exposed to the surrounding medium. Possibly, the greater ability to move accounts for the decreased dependence of growth on cell density.

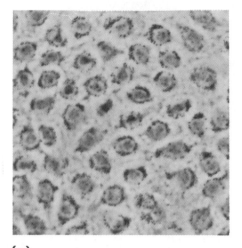 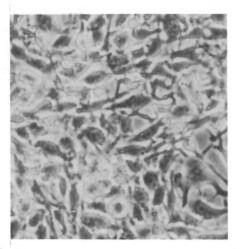

(a)   **(b)**

FIGURE 4-2   Micrographs showing confluent growth of (a) normal mouse 3T3 cells and (b) 3T3 cells transformed by polyoma virus. The transformed cells have a less regular shape and grow in a less organized way than normal cells. Blurred areas in the transformed culture are regions in which cells have piled up. (Courtesy of Walter Eckhart. From Freifelder, <u>Molecular Biology</u>, Jones and Bartlett.)

Decreased Serum Requirement of Cancer Cells

Growth of normal cells in culture requires the presence of a large number of organic substances in the medium. These substances, which are both small molecules and large proteins called <u>growth factors</u>, are normally supplied by the addition of fetal calf serum to the medium (serum is the liquid component of blood that remains after all cells have been removed). Cancer cells and cells transformed in culture are able to multiply in medium containing about 1/10 the usual concentration of serum. Some cancer and transformed cell lines will even grow in the absence of serum; such cells seem to make their own growth factors. It is not yet clear whether this is a general property of cancer cells, though the lack of a requirement for the usual serum concentration may be universal. More will be said about growth factors in a later section of this chapter.

Anchorage Independence

Most freshly isolated normal animal cells and cells obtained from cultures of normal cells will not grow when maintained in suspension in a liquid medium or embedded in a gel such as agar. As pointed out above, the cells normally find a surface to which they can attach and then spread and multiply (one exception is the white blood cell and related cells, which can grow in suspension). This type of growth, which is like that found in tissue, is called <u>anchorage-dependent growth</u>. Cells obtained from many tumors and cells transformed in culture by carcinogenic agents are able to grow quite well in suspension or in a gel. This mode of anchorage-independent growth can be used to isolate clones of cancer cells from mixtures. For example, a culture of normal cells can be treated with a carcinogen and then suspended in a gel: only the transformed cells will multiply, and each visible focus of growth consists of the progeny of a single transformed cell.

The physiology of anchorage dependence is not understood at all, though various hypotheses have been presented. One idea is that normal cells require cell-to-cell transfer of growth factors, so growth is poor when cells are physically separated from one another. Another explanation is based on the fact that normal cells flatten considerably on a surface, whereas transformed cells retain a more rounded shape. Possibly, the adsorption to a surface causes a stretching of the cell membrane that enables critical molecules, such as carrier molecules in the membrane to assume an optimal configuration for transport of nutrients and growth factors.

Anchorage dependence is an exceedingly important phenomenon in cancer biology. We mentioned earlier that all characteristics of transformed cells in culture are not necessarily required for tumor formation. By studying the tumor-forming ability of transformed cell lines that have lost any one of the properties just mentioned (density-independent growth, ability to grow without serum, or anchorage independence) it has been found that the one property observed in culture that is most closely associated with the ability to form tumors is anchorage independence. For example, with mouse cells, in which this phenomenon has been studied most carefully, loss of anchorage independence means loss of ability of injected cells to form a tumor in the mouse. Remembering the caution we have mentioned about generalizations in cancer biology, we must note that this correlation is not absolute; for example, in studying a series of cell lines isolated from human bladder cancers two cell lines grew in agar but were not tumorigenic, and one cell line failed to grow in agar but was tumorigenic.

Loss of the Restriction Point

In the description of the cell cycle in Chapter 2, it was pointed out that normal cells occasionally enter a quiescent state called G_0. The decision to enter G_0 or to continue in G_1 occurs at a point in G_1 called the <u>restriction point</u>. Once a cell passes this point, it must continue through S, G_2, and M and return to G_1. After this decision point, if progress of the cells through the cell cycle is inhibited in S, G_2, or M for any length of time, the cells die, as a result of release of numerous self-destructive enzymes from lysosomes. A variety of conditions, e.g., limitation of nutrients or growth factors, cause the normal cell to leave the cycle at the restriction point and enter the G_0 state; presumably, this is why normal cells terminate growth at high cell density and in medium containing little or no serum. In this state cells are unaffected by agents that would block DNA replication, mitosis, or progress through G_2, and hence cause death, so the decision to enter G_0 is a protective device. The biochemical mechanism of restriction point control is unknown. Most cancer cells and transformed cells lack this control, which accounts for their ability to continue to grow both to high cell densities and in the absence of serum. This lack of control is a potential weakness of cancer cells and is believed to be the reason for the killing effect of anticancer drugs that block cells in S, G_2, and M. These drugs, which are widely used as therapeutic agents, kill growing cells (that is, those that have escaped growth restriction) but do not affect normal cells, which ordinarily are in the protected G_0 state. Unfortunately, any dividing cell, such as those that produce hair, the lining of the intestine, red blood cells, and white blood cells, are also killed by these agents.

The decision of a normal cell to enter G_0 when challenged by certain agents is the basis of new anticancer treatments, as will be seen in Chapter 13. For example, a substance that causes normal growing cells to be arrested at the restriction point and enter G_0 will not cause a cancer cell to enter G_0. Thus, treatment of a patient first with this substance followed a day or so later by a mitotic inhibitor should cause death of cancer cells but no death of the G_0-protected normal cells. Clinical treatments based on such regimens are being developed, but definitive results are not yet available.

BIOCHEMICAL DIFFERENCES BETWEEN NORMAL AND CANCER CELLS

A variety of substances influence the growth of cells in culture; some of these are simply nutrients or ions, and others are known as growth factors. In many cases, there are significant differences in the amounts of these factors present in normal and tumor tissue and in the magnitude of the response of normal and cancer cells to these factors in culture. These differences are the subject of this section.

Chalones

Proteins that have some inhibitory activity on the multiplication of normal cells, termed chalones, have been isolated from skin, lung, liver, bone marrow, lymph nodes, kidney, and uterine lining. In each case the chalones are synthesized by the cells in the tissue. The inhibition is fairly tissue-specific in that each chalone inhibits mitosis in cells in tissue from which it was isolated but often not in other tissue types (that is, a chalone from lung tissue inhibits division of lung cells much more than liver cells).

Cancer tissue contains a much lower concentration of chalones, often as little as 2% of that found in normal tissue. Possibly a significant defect in cancer cells is a decreased ability either to synthesize chalones or to respond to them. Several laboratories are currently examining the intriguing possibility that treatment of cancer cells with chalones might arrest their growth.

Cyclic AMP and Cyclic GMP

Cyclic AMP (cyclic adenosine monophosphate) is a molecule that participates in the regulation of a large number of different biochemical reactions. Its influence is so wide that entire books have been written about it. Some years ago it was found that cyclic AMP added to the culture medium reduces the growth of normal and cancer cells. Furthermore, a related substance, cyclic GMP (cyclic guanosine monophosphate), restricts growth, and it was suggested that cell proliferation is regulated by the ratio of these two substances. However, a great many experiments have shown that the phenomena are much more complicated than earlier suspected and that most of the observations apply only to particular cell types.

Two points can be made with certainty: (1) cyclic AMP does reduce the rate of division of some normal and some transformed cells in culture, and (2) the concentration of cyclic AMP is lower in some transformed cells than in normal cells. What is completely unclear is whether changes in cyclic AMP concentrations or the cellular responses to the substance account in any way for the properties of transformed cells. There are conceivable ways by which cyclic AMP could affect growth. For example, since cyclic AMP regulates the transport of nutrients such as glucose, amino acids, and phosphate into cells, cyclic AMP could act by controlling the availability of these substances to the cell. Furthermore, since substances that stimulate growth, such as hormones, may decrease cyclic AMP concentrations, which in turn increases the transport of nutrients into cells, it is possible that the lower cyclic AMP levels in transformed cells result in increased nutrient uptake and thereby facilitate growth to high cell densities. However, whether such growth would be unregulated is certainly unclear.

Nutrients and Ions

In the preceding section we saw that normal and cancer cells occasionally differ in their ability to make use of or to respond to nutrients and suggested that cyclic AMP may be important in this difference. Another explanation is based on the observation that cancer cells in culture take up nutrients such as amino acids and sugars at rates that are greatly increased over that exhibited by untransformed cells of the same type. One may hypothesize that such increased transport results from alteration of transport sites on or within the surface membrane of cancer cells. This notion has not yet been put to a rigorous experimental test.

A variety of metal ions are required for the growth of all living cells. The calcium ion is especially interesting in cancer biology, for the minimum concentration sufficient for cell division is much lower for transformed cells than for normal cells. Specifically, the phenomenon is exemplified by an experiment with normal chicken cells and virally transformed cells. Both normal and transformed cells were placed in a growth medium with the normal concentration of serum, but low in calcium. Both normal cells and cancer cells divided actively.

However, if the serum concentration was somewhat lower, the tumor cells divided actively, while the normal cells did not divide. This inability of the normal cells to grow was not the low-serum effect described earlier in this chapter for two reasons: (1) in this experiment the serum concentration was not low enough to cause that effect and (2) increasing the calcium concentration to normal amounts allowed the normal cells to grow actively. Since it seems unlikely that calcium, which is needed in many biochemical reactions, is not needed by cancer cells, the interpretation of the results is the following: a growth factor in the serum probably aids in the uptake of calcium from the growth medium, and cancer cells probably take it up faster than normal cells from a low-calcium medium when the serum factor is absent. This is speculation though. Unfortunately, how calcium participates in growth regulation is unknown.

Growth Factors

Many molecules that affect the growth of eukaryotic cells have been isolated. The growth factors are usually simple proteins synthesized in particular cells and can often be found in blood plasma. Most of the factors have a wide range of activity, though they are not general stimulants of growth, because they are not effective in all tissue. For example, the activity of pituitary growth hormone, which stimulates growth of cartilage, muscle, and adipose tissue, is mediated through factors, called <u>somatomedins</u>, found in serum. Fibroblast growth factor, which has been isolated from the pituitary of the cow, is a powerful growth stimulant for cultured fibroblast cells and with several steroid hormones will replace serum in some but not all cell lines. Interestingly, fibroblast growth factor does not affect the growth of fibroblasts that have been transformed by several different tumor viruses.

<u>Nerve growth factor</u> is a stimulant that may prove to be of interest in cancer biology. It is made in a variety of embryonic tissues (not nerve tissue) and stimulates the growth of nerve cells in newborn animals. It has been found to be made by several cultured cell lines, of which two, neuroblastoma and glioma, are cancer cells. Of special interest are human melanoma cells. These cells not only contain nerve growth factor but have surface receptors for the factor, which suggests that this type of cancer cell, which arises embryologically from the neural crest (Chapter 2), could stimulate its own growth.

<u>Epidermal growth factor</u> is another substance of interest to cancer biology. In cell culture it stimulates a wide variety of cell types, and it is involved in a large number of physiological effects that are not necessarily related to cell growth. It acts by binding to specific receptors on the cell surface, and most, if not all, epithelial cells or cells derived from ectoderm possess these receptors. Furthermore, the epidermal growth factor of humans is almost identical to that of the mouse, indicating that the protein evolved a very long time ago on the evolutionary scale. With respect to its role in cell growth, cells grown in the presence of epidermal growth factor continue to multiply after formation of a confluent monolayer; thus, they behave like a

transformed cell in that they lack density-dependent growth. This observation suggests that continued exposure to the factor might be responsible for the excessive growth of cells in most tumors that are of epithelial origin. In accord with this idea, certain transformed cell types produce a substance similar to epidermal growth factor that binds to the receptors on the cell surface. Thus, such cells might stimulate their own rampant growth, though there is as yet no evidence to support this idea. In Chapter 8 when oncogenes (cancer-causing genes) are discussed, we will see that a modified receptor for epidermal growth factor is the product of a particular oncogene.

Another potentially important growth factor is platelet-derived growth factor (PDGF), a protein released into serum from blood platelets. It is a growth promoter, though its activity is limited to certain mesodermal cells, for example, fibroblasts and the smooth muscle cells of arteries. Epithelial cells are unaffected. With cells that respond to PDGF it is required for entry into the S phase. Cells requiring PDGF to enter S usually also require the somatomedins to progress through G_1. Fibroblasts transformed with SV40 virus no longer require either PDGF or the somatomedins and hence will grow to high cell density in medium containing very little serum. Some human and mouse fibroblast cell lines transformed by various chemical carcinogens cause tumors and some do not. Those that do cause tumors have no need for PDGF, whereas those that do not cause tumors grow poorly in platelet-free media. Since we do not yet know how PDGF exerts its effect on normal cells, little can be said other than that it may be involved in some cancer. More about PDGF will be given in the next chapter, when an oncogene that makes a similar substance is described.

Sarcoma growth factor is a growth-stimulating factor produced by fibroblasts that have been transformed with mouse sarcoma viruses. This factor competes with epidermal growth factor for binding sites on the cell surface. Of greatest interest is its ability to promote anchorage-independent growth of normal cells and hence to make normal cells behave like cancer cells. The phenomenon is reversible in the sense that anchorage dependence and growth control of normal cells both return if the factor is removed. Thus, sarcoma growth factor seems to be a growth factor produced specifically by certain transformed cells and able to stimulate their growth. This observation raises the possibility that the conversion of normal cells to at least some types of cancer cells might simply result from the ability to synthesize sarcoma growth factor, which could enable the cells to overcome the systems in the host animal that regulate normal growth.

Factors Present in Virus-Transformed Cells

Cells transformed by tumor viruses usually manufacture particular proteins that become localized in the cell nucleus. The best-studied are the T antigens of SV40 and polyoma viruses. These proteins cause initiation of DNA synthesis in cells transformed by these viruses. We will discuss the T antigens in a later chapter when viral transformation is described.

DIFFERENCES IN CELL SURFACES OF NORMAL AND CANCER CELLS

Animal cells are enclosed in membranes, whose inner regions determine, among other things, what molecules can enter and leave the cell, and whose surface contains a variety of chemical groups responsible for sensing the environment and receiving external molecular signals. The membrane and cell surface are involved in so many cellular activities that it comes as no surprise that differences have been observed between normal and cancer cells. From the point of view of cancer biology the membrane and cell surface are particularly important, since they seem to be involved in anchorage dependence, cell adhesion, and invasiveness through normal tissues. Table 4-1 lists most of the known differences. Some of these will be described in this chapter.

TABLE 4-1   Alterations commonly observed in cancer and transformed cells

Intracellular changes	Extracellular and environmental changes	Changes in growth habit
Gene alterations, activation, and repression	Increased protease	Decreased contact inhibition
Metabolic alterations	Increased nutrient uptake	Increased mobility
Unpolymerized cytoskeletal elements	Embryonic surface proteins	
Decreased production or response to chalones	Tumor-specific surface proteins	
Decreased amount of cyclic AMP, and increased amount of cyclic GMP	Decreased cell adhesion	
	Mobile lectin receptors	
	Increased lectin agglutinability	
	Decreased fibronectin	
	Incomplete sugar chains on various surface polymers	

Lectins

Lectins are a class of protein that bind to the sugars contained in particular carbohydrates. They have been isolated primarily from plants, though they have also been detected in bacteria, fungi, fish, snails, and some mammals. Their biological function is not known, and the principal interest in lectins has been as probes for the carbohydrates of cell surfaces. The two most commonly studied lectins are concanavalin A, which is obtained from the jack bean, and wheat germ agglutinin. Most lectins are multisubunit proteins (they consist of several identical protein molecules joined together), and each unit has a carbohydrate binding site (Figure 4-3). Because of the multiple binding sites, a total lectin unit can cause several particles to stick together, if each particle has a surface carbohydrate that can bind to the lectin. Since all cells have surface carbohydrates, lectins cause cells to clump (agglutinate). Lectins are of interest in the study of cancer, because most cancer cells are more easily agglutinated than normal cells (Figure 4-4). The specific observations are the following: (1) A variety of cells either obtained from tumors or transformed by viruses in culture form clumps at lectin concentrations that are too low to cause clumping of normal cells. (2) Cell lines that have been selected from transformed cell lines for having regained the property of density-dependent inhibition of growth have usually also lost the ability to be clumped by low concentrations of lectins. Similarly, cell lines that have been selected instead for loss of agglutinability by lectins also regain density-dependent growth and the requirement for high concentrations of serum (that is, their growth habit becomes normal).

The interpretation of the difference in sensitivity to lectins is that it reflects surface differences between normal cells and cancer cells. The most obvious explanation for agglutination by low concentrations of lectins is that cancer cells have more surface binding sites for lectins, but this is incorrect. The main difference seems to be that the binding sites on cancer cells are more mobile than those on normal cells. Also, as we will see, different carbohydrates are present on the two cell types, though this may not be especially significant with respect to lectin sensitivity.

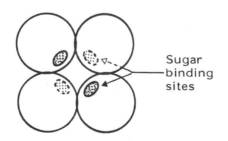

Sugar binding sites

FIGURE 4-3 A schematic diagram of a lectin that has four subunits and four binding sites for sugars.

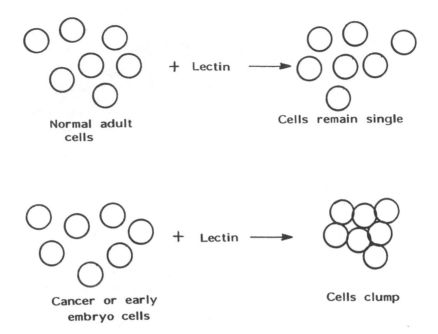

FIGURE 4-4   Diagram showing lectin-induced clumping of cancer cells and early embryo cells, but not of normal adult cells.

The mechanism of lectin-induced clumping has been elucidated from studies with lectins labeled with a fluorescent component (Figure 4-5). If normal cells are treated with fluorescent lectins and illuminated with near-ultraviolet light, one observes a faint fluorescence uniformly distributed over the cell surface. Thus, lectin-binding sites are located at a very large number of positions on the cell surface. When transformed cells or normal cells are used, again a faint fluorescence is seen on the cell surface. However, rather quickly the fluorescence appears to move until all fluorescence is concentrated in a single small region of the surface. This phenomenon, which is called capping, does not occur with normal cells and has the following explanation. The cell membrane of cancer cells is assumed to be quite fluid compared to that of normal cells, so lectin receptor sites are able to drift over the cell surface. (Recall from Chapter 2, Figure 2-7, that all membrane proteins can drift, but in normal cells this is a very slow process.) An individual lectin molecule will bind to a single surface receptor and then drift over the cell surface with the receptor. Since the lectin is multivalent, it will bind to a second receptor site, and the two receptors will drift together. Individual receptors are able to bind several different lectin molecules, so another lectin can bind, which can in turn bind still another receptor. The mutual linking continues until fairly soon all receptors and all bound lectins are in one region of the surface. Capping probably explains how lectins agglutinate

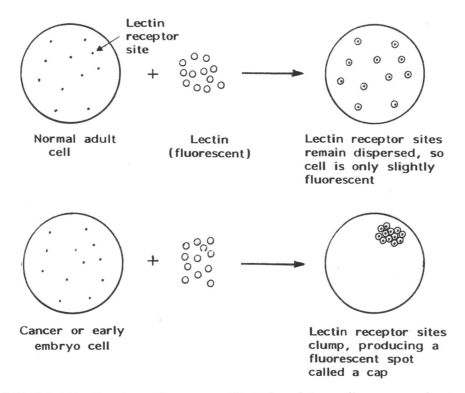

FIGURE 4-5 Capping of cancer cells induced by a fluorescent lectin. Normal adult cells do not exhibit capping.

cancer cells with greater efficiency than normal cells. That is, in the cap both lectins and lectin receptors are in a much higher concentration than when dispersed uniformly over the surface of a normal cell, thereby strengthening the cell-cell interactions for any given concentration of added lectin. It has been proposed that normal adult cells have cytoskeletal elements (microtubules and microfilaments) attached to the inner membrane surface, and these restrict the movement of the lectin receptor sites. Cancer cells, as will be seen, usually do not have organized cytoskeletal elements, which may account for the mobility of lectin receptors in their cell surfaces.

Many normal early embryonic cells also possess mobile cell surface lectin receptor sites and are also agglutinated by lectins. This is an example of what will be seen repeatedly, namely, a similarity between cancer cells and early embryonic cells.

Fibronectin

Fibronectin is a glycoprotein (protein with attached sugars) found on the surface of many types of normal nongrowing cells. It is loosely associated with the cell and forms a very thin fibrillar structure around and between cells. It also acts as an adhesive between some cell types and mediates the attachment of cultured cells to the cell culture vessels. For many cell types to grow in culture, fibronectin must be present in the serum; other cell types, which make their own fibronectin, do not require added fibronectin. Cancer cells and transformed cells have little or no fibronectin on their surfaces and adsorb poorly to the surface of the culture vessel; however, they continue to grow. Addition of fibronectin to cultures of some tumor cells causes normalization of cell adhesion, flattens cells, and restores contact inhibition of cell movement. However, it does not normalize growth control: cells still grow in small amounts of serum, and lack density-dependent growth and anchorage dependence. Fibronectin is found on the surface of cells of benign tumors and very early primary carcinomas, but is totally lacking on highly malignant and metastatic tumors. Thus, it is believed that loss of fibronectin may correlate not with rampant growth but with ability to spread throughout the body.

Some evidence exists that fibronectin is still synthesized in some types of cancer cells but is rapidly shed from the cell surface due to excessive production of enzymes that degrade proteins and carbohydrates (see later section on enzymes that degrade proteins).

Recent evidence also suggests that fibronectin may be connected to bundles of microfilaments inside the cell and may help cells flatten and adhere to culture surfaces. These microfilaments may play a role in keeping cells in a stabilized, controlled growth pattern. Drugs such as cytochalasin, which cause breakdown of bundles of microfilaments, also cause release of fibronectin from the cell surface.

Adhesion

In the next chapter, we will consider how tumor cells spread through the body, that is, the metastatic process. The initial step in metastasis is the separation of a tumor cell from the tumor mass. In order to understand this process, we must examine the nature of cell adhesion and the decrease of adhesion that is characteristic of many cancer cells. Adhesion has been studied for many years, and unfortunately it is still not understood clearly. However, what seems clear is that cell adhesion is determined by cell surface carbohydrates. A variety of models of cell adhesion have been proposed; each depends heavily on details of the biochemistry of synthesis of the cell surface sugars and will not be described here. All of the models seem to have some support from experimental results, but also there are always results that disagree with the models; thus, our understanding of adhesion is still incomplete. The most certain statement that can be made is that the surface carbohydrates of normal and cancer cells differ; substances found on cancer cells are not found on normal cells (though some are found on embryonic cells), and substances found on normal cells are not always found on cancer cells.

We will not go into any details about the chemical differences, but a general statement can be made. Most surface carbohydrates are made by a series of biochemical changes, and it has been observed that transformed cells generally possess incomplete carbohydrate chains on their surfaces. Many enzymes are involved in the synthetic reactions on the surface. One class is called glycosyl transferases, and transformed cells have reduced amounts of these enzymes. Some schools of thought, which believe that the enzymes themselves participate in cell adhesion, consider the small amount of the enzymes to be important in the low adhesion between cancer cells. There is some experimental support for this notion, but it is far from being unambiguous.

Virus-Induced and Embryonic Antigens on the Cell Surface

Many of the proteins and glycoproteins on the cell surface are detected by immunological tests and hence are commonly referred to as surface antigens. When cells are transformed by viruses, new molecules form on the surface. Those that are not found on any normal cell are called tumor-specific antigens. The antigens are usually determined by the virus in that the same antigen is found in different cell types transformed by the same virus. The situation is quite different with cells transformed by chemical carcinogens or radiation; the tumor antigens formed in these cells do not depend upon the agent used, but vary with cell type.

In addition to tumor-specific antigens, many induced and naturally occurring tumor cells containing embryonic antigens (Figure 4-6). These antigens, which are present in embryonic tissues, are not found in normal adult tissues. Note that this means that embryonic antigens disappear as cells mature and differentiate, and often reappear when the adult cells become transformed into cancer cells. This observation, plus others that we have mentioned earlier, has given rise to the idea that production of a cancer cell may, in some cases, simply be a reversion to the embryonic state of the cells. That is, some carcinogenesis may involve reactivation of genes that were active in embryonic life but were turned off in the normal adult life of the cells. Two of the more commonly observed embryonic antigens are the following: alpha-fetoprotein, found in cancer of the liver (hepatomas), testis, pancreas, and gastrointestinal tract; and carcinoembryonic antigen (CEA) found in cancer of the gastrointestinal tract, pancreas, liver, and lung.

The embryonic and tumor-specific antigens may cause the host to produce antibodies against the antigens. We will return to the possible immune response against cancer in Chapter 9.

A third class of surface antigens consists of antigens present in normal adult cells but in a hidden state. That is, they are covered by other surface molecules and are therefore inaccessible to immunological tests. In transformed cells these antigens are frequently exposed.

In Chapters 12 and 13 we will see that surface antigens may be the key to new approaches in therapy, detection, and prevention of some cancers.

PROTEIN-DEGRADING ENZYMES AND CANCER CELLS

The final aspect of altered cancer cell surfaces to be considered here

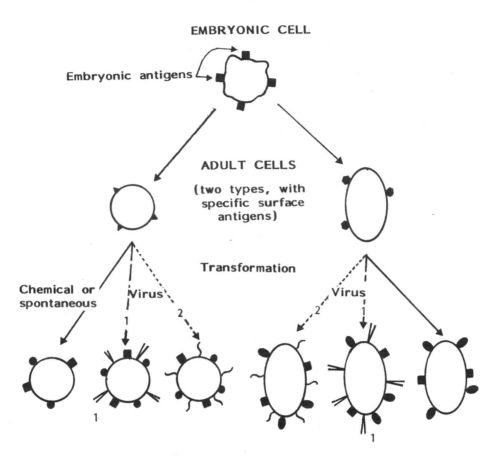

EMBRYONIC CELL

Embryonic antigens

ADULT CELLS

(two types, with specific surface antigens)

Transformation

Chemical or spontaneous

Virus

Virus

TRANSFORMED CELLS

with cell-type-specific (●, ◕), virus-specific (∫, ◁), and embryonic (■) surface antigens

FIGURE 4-6 Diagram showing the various surface antigens present on embryonic, adult, and transformed cells. Embryonic antigens are no longer made by adult cells, but some of them reappear on transformed cells. If the cell is transformed by a virus, viral antigens may also be present.

is the presence of many proteolytic (protein-degrading) enzymes. In Chapter 2 we mentioned that many types of cancer cells show increased levels of these enzymes and that this may be related to the invasive properties of tumor cells. This characteristic of cancer cells, because of its probable importance in causing altered cell behavior, will now be examined in more detail.

A variety of protein-degrading enzymes (proteases) are excreted by many cancer cells. One of the most commonly observed is called plasminogen activator. The production of plasminogen activator goes hand in hand with transformation in culture (by viruses, radiation, and chemical carcinogens) of a large number of cell lines. At one time it was thought that the presence of this protein could be used as an absolute assay for cancer cells. However, some cancer cells do not secrete plasminogen activator and a variety of normal cells do. Nonetheless the phenomenon is considered to be important in cancer biology. What seems likely is that the proteases are involved in invasiveness of surrounding tissue rather than transformation itself. That is, production of these enzymes may degrade sufficient intracellular protein to break down cell adhesion between tumor cells and allow cells from a primary tumor to leave the tumor mass. In addition, by dissolving away proteins in normal cells, individual tumor cells can invade normal tissue and establish new foci of growth.

Some evidence also exists that the surface proteases may participate in early stages of tumor formation. For example, cultured mouse melanoma cells are able to produce tumors when injected in another mouse. However, if cell lines are selected that produce much less plasminogen activator, the cells lose their ability to form tumors. In addition, general inhibitors of proteases inhibit the growth of some transformed cell lines in culture and restore density-dependent growth regulation to other transformed cell lines. Also, if some types of normal cells are treated with proteases, they undergo a burst of cell division and temporarily resemble tumor cells. Many normal cells treated with proteases become agglutinable with lectins, suggesting that the mobility of cell surface receptor sites is increased. This increased mobility of receptor sites may be due to direct action of the proteases at the cell surface or be caused by the breakdown of cytoskeletal elements such as microtubules and microfilaments. Such cytoskeletal elements in normal cells are degraded when the cells are treated with these enzymes, and this breakdown may release surface receptors that are anchored by microtubules.

There is indirect evidence that proteases are released into the blood stream by malignant tumors. The principal observation is the presence of fragments of normal blood proteins in the blood of patients with highly malignant cancer. Presumably these fragments result from degradation of the proteins by the excessive amount of the enzymes. Research is in progress to see whether detection of minute quantities of these fragments could be used as a diagnostic tool for early detection of cancer.

DIFFERENCES IN THE CYTOSKELETON OF NORMAL AND CANCER CELLS

Recall from Chapter 2 that normal cells usually have an extensive and well-organized cytoskeleton consisting of bundles of microfilaments and microtubules. These structures consist of polymerized subunits of specific proteins. Cancer cells in culture possess the subunits, but usually in the unpolymerized state (Figure 4-7). In other words, cancer cells generally contain the building blocks of the microfilaments, but not the organized microfilaments themselves.

During mitosis normal cells also exhibit altered cytoskeletons in that microfilaments and microtubules usually break down to the individual protein subunits. Since the cytoskeleton probably helps to maintain the shape of normal cells and tissue patterns and may maintain specific membrane functions and receptors, the depolymerized state of cytoskeletal elements in normal dividing cells and in cancer cells is consistent with the observed rounding up and lack of adhesion of dividing cells.

The cause of the depolymerized state of the cytoskeleton in cancer cells is unknown; a variety of reasons have been suggested, but none have been proved. Some new work suggests that cancer cells have a lowered pH and that this may be the key factor in preventing polymerization. Actin, the building block of microfilaments, does not polymerize when the pH drops below 7.0.

ALTERATIONS IN CELLULAR BIOCHEMISTRY

The biochemistry of cancer cells often varies from one type of cancer to another. There are volumes of observations on the differences and similarities in metabolism of cancer cells and normal cells, but not many generalizations can be made. Some metabolic pathways, such as those utilized in DNA synthesis, are usually more active in cancer cells. However, this is probably an accompaniment to transformation rather than a cause.

Another biochemical observation whose significance has been considered at different times to be either exceedingly important or quite unimportant is the fact that cancer cells are better able to

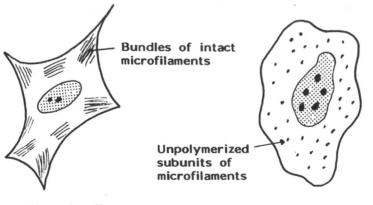

Bundles of intact microfilaments

Unpolymerized subunits of microfilaments

Normal cell   Cancer cell

FIGURE 4-7 Schematic diagram of a normal cell and a transformed cell showing how the shape of a normal cell is determined by the presence of bundles of microfilaments. The microfilament subunits do not polymerize in transformed cells, which therefore are rounder.

metabolize glucose in the absence of oxygen than are normal cells. At the present time, this is considered to be unrelated to the actual conversion from normal to cancer cells but merely something that occurs in the development of certain tumors. It is reflected in an increased ability to survive in the absence of oxygen, and perhaps it is what enables tumors to reach a particular size before it becomes necessary for capillaries to penetrate the tumor and supply oxygen. Anaerobic metabolism of glucose produces acid (decreases intracellular pH); thus, it has been suggested that such metabolism is responsible for the lack of polymerization of the cytoskeleton, which does not occur at acid pH, as mentioned in the previous section.

Many enzymes exist in several forms at various stages of development of the organism. For example, there may be forms characteristic of particular tissues, or, more interesting from the point of view of cancer biology, differences between embryonic, fetal, and adult forms. Again, few generalizations can be made, but the forms of many enzymes in cancer cells often resemble those of fetal tissue rather than those of the adult tissue from which the tumor is derived. This is another example of the possible return of normal cells to a less differentiated embryonic state in the transformation process.

ADDITIONAL READINGS

Alberts, B., D. Bray, J. Lewis, M. Raff, K. Roberts, and J.D. Watson. 1983. Molecular Biology of the Cell. Chapters 10, 12. Garland.

Freifelder, D. 1983. Molecular Biology. Chapter 21. Jones and Bartlett.

Ruddon, R.W. 1981. Cancer Biology. Chapter 5. Oxford.

5

Cellular Basis of Invasion and Metastasis

Normal tissues consist of cells that are in organized, stable arrays. Cell division, if it occurs at all, is usually confined to a specific region of the tissue, and daughter cells remain within the parent tissue. A tumor differs from normal tissue in that the cells are typically disorganized and cell division occurs in all regions of the tumor mass. The key feature of a tumor that is malignant is that the tumor cells spread beyond the confines of the tissue of origin. How this occurs is the topic of this chapter.

OUTLINE OF THE MOVEMENT OF TUMOR CELLS: SOME DEFINITIONS

A primary tumor is a tumor mass present at the site of initial conversion of a normal cell to a tumor cell. If all cells remained in the primary tumor, cancer would be of little importance. Growth of the tumor would produce pressure on surrounding tissue, which would ultimately be deleterious, but the well-defined tumor mass could be excised by surgery in a straightforward and permanent way. However, tumor cells do not always remain at the primary site, but move away by one of two processes: (1) invasion, or the movement of cells into neighboring space occupied by other tissues; and (2) metastasis, the spread of cells to distant sites, usually via the bloodtream, lymphatic system, or through body spaces. Substantial invasion usually occurs before any metastasis takes place.

Invasion in its simplest form is merely the expansion of tumor cells into surrounding tissues as a result of continuous division of cancer cells. However, active cell movement may also occur. Cells in malignant cancers tend to adhere poorly to each other, break away from the tumor mass, and then move away from each other by actual movement of the cell (akin to the movement of an amoeba). Such movement does not occur in normal tissue. Normal cells do indeed move both in culture and in the course of embryological development, but when normal adult cells in culture touch each other, they usually stop both growth and movement, as we have seen in Chapter 4. However, cancer cells, at least in culture, are not controlled by cell contact, and in the body they continue to grow and move into surrounding tissues. Also, most cancer cells release proteases (enzymes that degrade proteins), which probably help them digest away surrounding tissue materials, thereby facilitating invasion.

Metastasis is the spread of tumor cells to areas not directly adjacent to the primary tumor. Such spread can occur by invasion of blood or lymph vessels or by penetration of the cancer cells into the body cavity or spaces surrounding organs.

Metastasis generally occurs in several stages (Figure 5-1):

1. Detachment of cells from the primary tumor.
2. Migration of tumor cells, penetration (invasion) of these cells into lymph vessels or blood vessels, and dissemination of the cells or cell clusters to distant areas.
3. Lodging of tumor cells in blood vessels of distant organs.
4. Invasion of tumor cells through the vessel walls and into the tissue of secondary sites.
5. Growth of secondary tumors at the secondary sites.

The first stage, detachment of cells from the primary tumor (Figure 5-2), is probably a result of a change in the adhesive properties of the cells. Without cell detachment from the primary tumor, metastasis could not occur. In order to be able to think about this change it

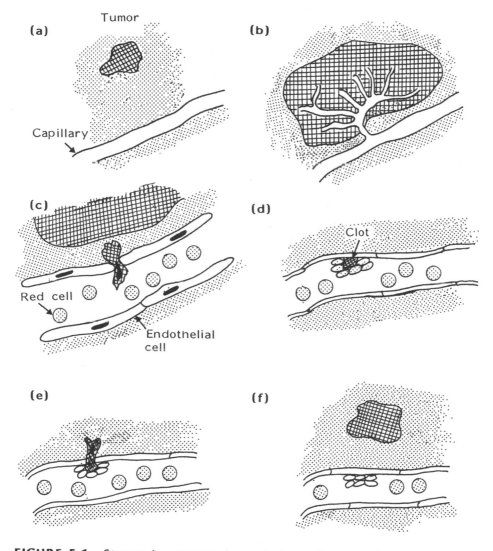

FIGURE 5-1 Stages in metastasis. (a) A small tumor forms. (b) New capillaries grow into tumor, enabling tumor to enlarge. (c) A tumor cell breaks loose from the tumor mass and passes between the endothelial cells of the capillary wall. (d) The cell is carried through the blood stream until it is trapped in a clot. (e) Cell passes out of the capillary into surrounding tissue. (f) Secondary tumor develops.

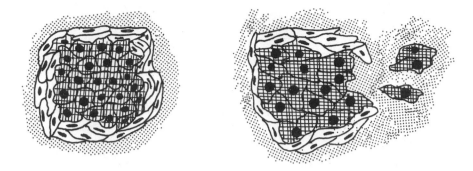

FIGURE 5-2   An early step in invasion. Left panel: a small tumor (shaded cells) forms, often surrounded by a capsule of nontumor cells (unshaded cells). Right panel: tumor cells detach from the tumor mass and migrate into the surrounding tissue (stippled area).

is necessary to understand something about the nature of cell-cell adhesion. Ideally one would like to study this phenomenon with normal cells and cancer cells, but as we will see in the next section, a great deal of rather fundamental information has been obtained from more elementary experiments with simple organisms and embryonic tissues. We begin with some key experiments with sponges; later we will relate these observations to cancer.

CELL ADHESION

Sponges, which are fairly simple multicellular marine animals, can be disaggregated into single cells merely by forcing the animal through silk cloth. When these separated sponge cells are allowed to settle in a dish of sea water, they drift around, seemingly at random, stick to one another, and ultimately form a new sponge. If cells from a species of red sponge are mixed with cells from a species of purple sponge, the red cells aggregate only with other red cells and form a red sponge, while the purple cells form a purple sponge (Figure 5-3). Thus, recognition of sponge cells is species-specific. This observed specificity has served as a model system to study adhesive recognition in other systems.

An initial question that was asked about the specificity was whether it occurred because a cell preferentially migrated on the bottom of the container to another cell of the same species, or if the adhesion itself was species-specific. This question was answered by placing the mixture of single cells in a rotary stirrer; with continual stirring cells would not fall to the bottom and collisions between both kinds of cells would occur. In this experiment it was observed that, when rotated together, red and purple sponge cells still formed aggregates consisting mainly of only one type of cell: red stuck to red, and purple stuck to purple. Thus, the reason for species-specific aggregation is that each type of cell preferentially sticks to its own kind.

In a second experiment the molecular nature of the species-specific adhesion of sponge cells was investigated. In this experiment it was found that sponges could also be disaggregated to yield single cells by immersing the animal in sea water from which calcium and magnesium had been removed. These cells, would reaggregate if the calcium and magnesium were added back to the liquid used to separate to the cells. However, they would not reaggregate when placed in fresh sea water, suggesting that something is present in the water used during disaggregation but absent in the fresh sea water; that is, some factor had been released to the fluid when the sponges disaggregated. To test whether the factor was species-specific, the cells were removed from the original fluid and then added to the fluid used in the

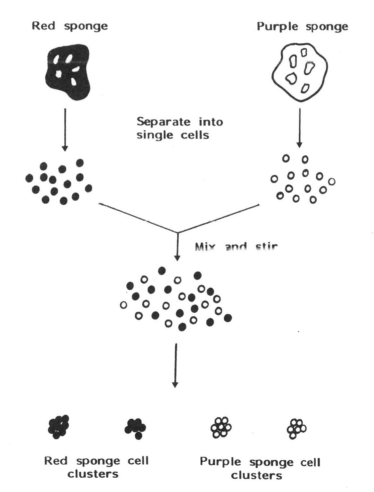

FIGURE 5-3 An experiment with disaggregated sponges that showed that only like cells can reaggregate. See text for details.

disaggregation, plus calcium. That is, red sponge cells were mixed with the fluid obtained by disaggregating purple sponges (plus calcium), and purple cells were added to the fluid obtained by disaggregating red sponges (plus calcium). In neither case did aggregation occur: fluid from the purple sponges promoted aggregation only of purple sponge cells, and fluid from the red sponges caused aggregation only of red sponge cells (Figure 5-4). It was concluded from this experiment that a molecule responsible for species-specific adhesion was released into the fluid when the sponge was disaggregated. Restoration of these molecules to the cells in the presence of calcium enabled the cells to rejoin. The adhesion-promoting molecules (adhesion factors) were then purified and found to be proteins to which carbohydrates are linked (glycoproteins), the same class of molecules on the surface of most cells that also participate in cell adhesion. Many glycoproteins that promote adhesion have been isolated and characterized, but the nature of the bond between readhering sponge cells is not yet known.

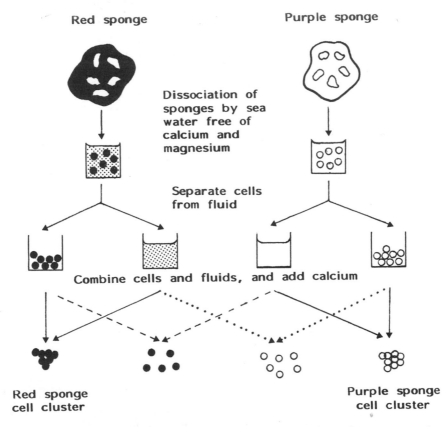

FIGURE 5-4 An experiment with sponge cells that demonstrated the existence of species-specific cell adhesion factors. See text for details.

The methods used in studying sponge cell adhesion have also been used to study adhesion of embryonic cells. Embryos of all types can be disaggregated into single cells using solutions that are either alkaline, free of calcium and magnesium, or containing proteolytic enzymes such as trypsin. Disaggregated cells from either the whole embryo or a variety of embryonic tissues first form disordered aggregates containing many types of cells. However, the cells are not tightly bound to one another, and they either separate or move through the aggregate. After a day or two, the cells tend to become sorted into groups of only one or a small number of cell type. In general, cells seek their own kind, and the mixed cell aggregate becomes transformed into an aggregate containing several areas composed of only one cell type. For example, retina cells stick to retina cells, and pre-heart cells stick to pre-heart cells. How sorting occurs is unclear, but it appears to occur by a continual loosening and strengthening of intercellular bonds, modulated by the relative strengths of adhesiveness between the different cell types: the most tightly adhesive cells ultimately squeeze together towards the center of the aggregate, with the less adhesive cells migrating to the periphery. Recently, it has been found that if embryos are disaggregated in certain ways, the released cells behave like sponge cells in that cells of a particular type immediately adhere only to other cells of the same type.

In the sponge experiments we saw that specific adhesion factors could be isolated. Such molecules have also been isolated from embryonic cells. For example, a molecule isolated from the culture medium in which chick embryo neural retina cells were grown promotes adhesiveness of embryonic neural retina cells but not of cells from other embryonic organs. The size of the aggregate also depends on the amount of the adhesion factor added to the cells.

ADHESION OF CANCER CELLS

In 1944 an important set of experiments was carried out that showed that cells in primary tumors are less adhesive to one another than normal cells of the same type and that this defect could lead to spread of cancer. In these experiments the mechanical force required to separate pairs of tumor cells and pairs of normal cells was measured by inserting a microneedle in each cell and recording the force needed to pull the cells apart. The force required to pull cancer cells apart was less than that needed to pull apart normal cells of the same tissue.

A variety of experiments have suggested explanations for the reduced adhesiveness of cancer cells. It is known that many tissues can be disaggregated merely by removing calcium from the fluid (as we saw with the sponges). Analysis of the cells used in the microneedle experiments of the preceding paragraph showed that the cancer cells usually contained about half the amount of calcium than did the normal cells from the same tissue. It has been suggested that the low calcium concentration is an important factor in the weaker adhesion of cancer cells; however, there is little proof at present for such a conclusion. Another explanation is based upon the high levels of surface proteolytic enzymes found in many cancer cells. Since incubation of almost any tissue in a medium containing proteases effectively separates the tissues into single cells by dissolving the adhesion proteins, the excessive amounts of protease on the surfaces of cancer cells could easily weaken the adhesive strength.

Some tumor cells, for instance, mouse ascites cells, do not adhere at all and exist as cell suspensions in the body. These cells are not adhesive because they do not synthesize cell surface carbohydrates required for cell adhesion. If these cells are supplied with the amino acid, L-glutamine, they become more adhesive (Figure 5-5). A variety

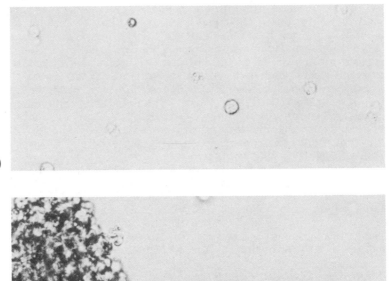

(a)

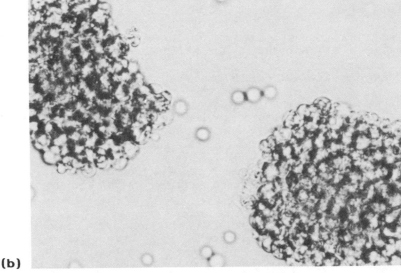

(b)

FIGURE 5-5 Demonstration that mouse ascites tumor cells require L-glutamine for aggregation. (a) No L-glutamine. (b) With L-glutamine. Most normal cells do not require added L-glutamine for adhesion; mouse ascites cells probably have a defect in either synthesis, transport, or storage of L-glutamine.

of experiments suggested that L-glutamine was used by the cells to synthesize a key intermediate in the formation of the cell surface carbohydrates required for adhesion. Studies of cultured mouse teratoma cells indicate that the cells become more adhesive when activity levels of the enzyme glutamine synthetase increase in these cells. These results suggest that the altered adhesiveness of these cells may result from decreased ability to synthesize L-glutamine. Defective storage or transport of this amino acid may also play a role in the apparent need for an extra supply of this amino acid for adhesion in these cells.

Recall that cancer cells often exhibit incomplete surface carbohydrate chains and possibly lowered levels of glycosyl transferase activity at their cell surfaces. Considering what we have said (Chapters 2 and 4) about the potential role of carbohydrates and glycosyl transferases in cell adhesion, we may speculate that synthesis of incomplete surface carbohydrates and lowered levels of surface glycosyl transferase activity may play a role in the reduced adhesiveness of cells in primary tumors.

We pointed out in Chapter 2 that the shape of cells is determined by the cytoskeleton and that cancer cells synthesize less fibronectin and, as a result, tend to round up. This tendency puts tension on the cell membrane, perhaps sufficient to weaken adhesive forces. Thus, it is possible that as a tumor develops, fibronectin synthesis becomes reduced as new cells form, until cells are produced that adhere only weakly to the tumor mass. This sequence of events, if it in fact occurs, could be responsible for the separation of cells from the main body of large tumors.

MIGRATION AND DISSEMINATION OF CANCER CELLS

When cells separate from a primary tumor, they may form nearby clusters of tumor cells or, of much greater significance for the survival of the organism, they may invade blood and lymph vessels and become disseminated to secondary sites in the body. It is not known with certainty whether the outcomes, nearby invasion versus dissemination by blood and lymph, are just happenstance. However, there is some evidence that suggests that the migratory characteristics of some invasive and metastatic cancer cells may result from specific factors given off by the cells themselves. When a portion of a layer of normal cells in culture is scraped off the surface on which the cells are growing and then removed from the culture vessel, the cells do not migrate into the cleared area if serum is absent from the medium. However, if the same treatment is given to a layer of malignant cells in culture, cells will migrate into a scraped area in serum-free medium. A "migration factor" can be isolated from the culture of malignant cells that will stimulate normal cells to migrate in a serum-free medium (Figure 5-6). Such a factor may stimulate cells in tumors to migrate away from the primary tumor. This phenomenon is obviously a field of active research.

The ability of cancer cells to penetrate blood and lymph vessels may be associated with the migratory ability of cancer cells. Such invasiveness also may be related to lack of contact inhibition of cell

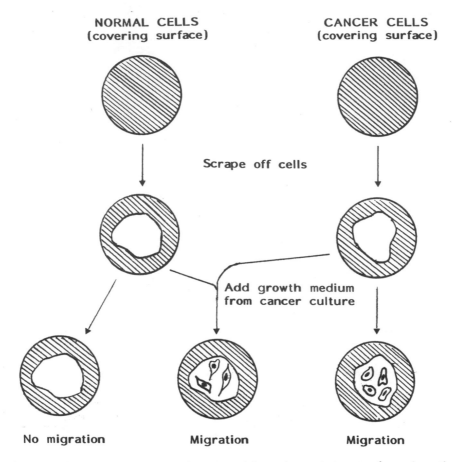

NORMAL CELLS
(covering surface)

CANCER CELLS
(covering surface)

Scrape off cells

Add growth medium
from cancer culture

No migration   Migration   Migration

FIGURE 5-6 An experiment demonstrating the existence of a migration factor in cancer cell cultures. Fluid from a scraped culture of cancer cells stimulates normal cells to migrate into the scraped area of a normal culture.

movement of various cancer cells observed in culture. As we have seen in Chapter 4, not only does cell-cell contact inhibit growth of normal cells in culture, but it also inhibits their movement. However, transformed cells in culture do not stop migrating when in contact with each other. If cancer cells in the body share these characteristics, then the ability to migrate through blood vessels may result in part from the lack of signals that normally tell the cells to stop migrating.

We have mentioned several times that proteases are often excluded from cancer cell surfaces and that these proteases may be important in determining whether a tumor can grow into the surrounding tissue. Some evidence for a role of proteases in causing release of cells from a tumor mass has been obtained. For example, treatment of an isolated tumor with pepstatin A, a protease inhibitor, increased the adhesiveness of tumor cells and blocked disaggregation of tumor cell clusters. These enzymes probably also participate in the erosion of blood vessel walls during metastatic spread. It is also possible that invasion of blood vessels by cancer cells is sometimes the result of pressure produced by the expanding tumor. High tissue pressure can force tumor fragments through a damaged blood vessel into the blood stream. However, this means of penetration is mechanical and is not due to any special properties of the individual cancer cells.

Invasive behavior and penetration of blood vessels is not restricted to cancer cells. For example, the placenta "metastasizes" towards the end of pregnancy in the sense that placenta cells can be found in the circulation of the mother. However, this has no lasting effects, since hormonal changes at birth probably kill the remaining disseminated placenta cells. Cells that give rise to pigment cells, the melanoblasts, migrate actively through tissues of embryos, but eventually home to specific sites where they differentiate into pigment cells. Also, many white blood cells exit and enter the blood vessels in their quest for attacking foreign invaders in the tissues and circulation. Clearly, the ability to migrate and invade blood vessels is not restricted to malignant cells. This invasive behavior must be coupled with uncontrolled cell growth for the truly malignant state to emerge.

SURVIVAL OF METASTASIZING CELLS

Migration of cancer cells throughout the body is not sufficient to cause distant tumors, because the cells must be able to survive environmental conditions different from those of the tissue of origin. Blood and lymph, which provide the major means of transport of cancer cells, are hostile environments for cells not adapted to live there, and only about 1 percent of cancer cells in the circulation survive to form secondary tumors. Most of the cells either die in the blood stream or reach the lung where they are either destroyed or lie dormant, possibly for many years. It is thought that blood serum contains waste products and other substances that are toxic to the cancer cells. If so, one may ask how any of them survive and colonize distant sites. It is considered likely that survivors are derived from small clusters of cancer cells that enter the bloodstream; the inner cells in the clusters are presumably protected from the hostile environmental conditions.

SITE SELECTION AND DEVELOPMENT OF SECONDARY TUMORS

The final stages in metastatic tumor spread involve the arrest of cancer cells at secondary sites and growth of these cells into secondary tumors. Although the causes of arrest of cancer cells and the means by which they establish themselves at certain sites are not clearly understood, some facets of the problem are being elucidated. One fact that stands out is derived from autopsies of individuals who died of metastatic cancer: some sites frequently have tumors, whereas other sites are almost always free of tumors. For example, liver, lungs, lymph nodes, adrenal glands, brain, and vertebral bone marrow are common sites of secondary tumors, whereas spleen, heart, and skeletal muscle are seldom affected. Thus, it is clear that some sort of selectivity must exist in the development of secondary cancers. We shall discuss this feature of metastasis after describing how cells manage to move from a primary site to a secondary site.

There are basically two mechanisms for spread of cancer cells. One, direct extension of tumor cells into the body cavity, is fairly easy to understand. For example, lung cancer cells can slough off the surface of the tumor and directly enter the pleural cavity. Ovarian cancer cells can shed cells into the peritoneal cavity, and brain cancers can release cells to the cerebrospinal fluid. With these tumors the secondary sites are generally determined by simple geometric effects. (In some instances, a surgeon may inadvertently cause tumor spread during removal of a primary tumor. Cancer cells may be picked up on surgical instruments and spread to other regions in the surgical field. Surgeons, however, are keenly aware of this problem and take special care to prevent transfer of tumor cells to other regions of the body.) Spreading of tumor cells through the blood and lymph is a more complicated process and many questions remain unanswered. The most informative studies of the actual process of spreading were those in which windows were constructed in the ears of rabbits. In these experiments tumor cells stained with a colored dye that made them identifiable were injected into small arteries of the ear, and the events that occurred were recorded on film. The following sequence of events was observed. Within minutes after injection of the tumor cells, the cells adhered firmly to the inner wall of a capillary (the capillary endothelium). A clot formed and other cells became trapped in the clot. By 24 hours the cancer cells had begun to divide. In a way that is not clear, but perhaps a result of secretion of proteolytic enzymes, the capillary wall became visibly damaged. Then, white blood cells in the capillaries penetrated the damaged area, followed by tumor cells. Finally, the cancer cells continued to grow, nearly obliterating the capillaries. Once the tumor had reached a critical size, new capillaries grew into this area of the dividing tumor, after which a large secondary tumor developed (Figure 5-1). Although filming was only performed in the ear, secondary tumors arose in numerous parts of the body of the rabbit. Whether the sequence of events is the same throughout the body is not known, but it is widely believed that the processes are at least similar.

In the course of this filming an important experiment was carried out that shed some light on one aspect of the sequence. Anticoagulants (substances that prevent formation of clots) were administered shortly after injection of the tumor cells. As a result, clots did not form, and the number of secondary tumors produced in the rabbits was significantly reduced. It is not known whether the clot that forms around the tumor cells in the capillaries serves to protect the cancer cells and instead enables them to invade the capillary walls, or if it has another function. Possibly, it may serve as a network on which the white blood cells can migrate and help to damage the capillary endothelium.

Note that after a secondary tumor becomes established, the capillary bed through which the cells initially passed from the blood stream to the tissue is destroyed. Without a constant supply of nutrients and of oxygen the tumor cells are unable to multiply indefinitely, and the maximum size of such growth is probably not much more than a few millimeters across. Continued growth requires development of new blood vessels (vascularization) in the tumor. In the films new capillaries were observed to grow into tumors at the rapid rate of up to 1 millimeter each day. The signal to form capillaries is a complex protein-containing molecular aggregate produced by the tumor cells. This molecular aggregate is called tumor angiogenesis factor. A variety of such factors have been isolated from different tumors and, interestingly, from placental tissue. One approach that is being taken to elicit cures for cancer is the development of antagonists of this factor.

We mentioned above that there is an apparent site selectivity in the formation of secondary tumors: primary tumors in certain organs tend to metastasize to preferred sites (Table 5-1). For example, breast adenocarcinoma most frequently metastasizes to the regional lymph nodes and then to liver, lungs, bones, ovaries, and adrenal glands; lung cancers frequently metastasize to the brain; prostate cancers often metastasize to the bones of the spine, and stomach adenocarcinomas metastasize to the regional lymph nodes and then to the liver and lungs. There are two reasons for this selectivity: (1) the relative geometry of the primary and secondary sites and (2) selective stickiness. The first is fairly easy to understand. For

TABLE 5-1   Metastatic routes for various primary cancers

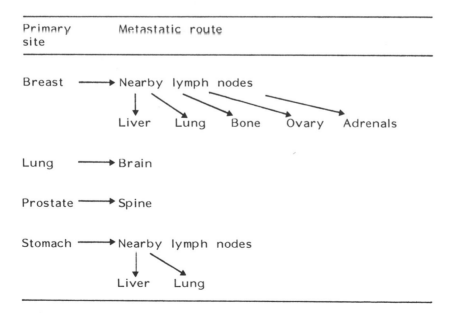

Primary site	Metastatic route

Breast ⟶ Nearby lymph nodes → Liver Lung Bone Ovary Adrenals

Lung ⟶ Brain

Prostate ⟶ Spine

Stomach ⟶ Nearby lymph nodes → Liver Lung

example, the body contains natural channels such as the veins and lymph system and spaces around muscles and nerves, so cancer cells that have left a primary tumor may simply become lodged in the first available place. For example, carcinomas of the breast, stomach, colon, and lung most frequently metastasize to regional (nearby) lymph nodes, and small veins from the prostate to bone easily account for the tendency of prostatic cancer to move to bone.

In many cases, the secondary sites cannot be accounted for by simple geometry, and selective adhesion is probably the critical point. Two experiments suggest this possibility. In one experiment tumor cells were obtained by disaggregation of tumors and then mixed with single cells from a variety of tissues (Figure 5-7). It was found that adhesion did not occur at random, but specific cells paired. For example, cells of melanomas from several individuals stuck better to lung cells than to any other cell type. Indeed, the lung is the site in which most secondary tumors develop from the line of melanoma used in the experiments. Melanomas from a few individuals selectively stuck to brain, adrenal, and ovary cells and selectively colonized

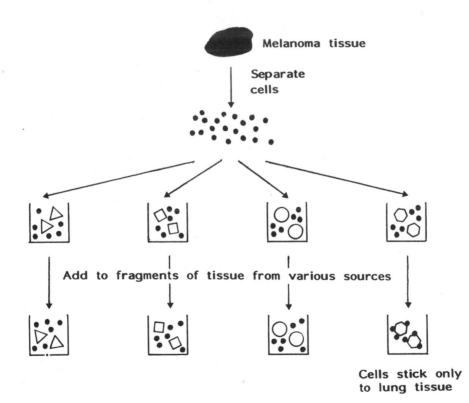

FIGURE 5-7   Diagram showing that cells obtained from a single melanoma selectively adhere to lung tissue.

these organs when injected into an animal. In another series of experiments it was shown that the tendency to metastasize to a particular site could be increased by selection. In this experiment a mouse melanoma cell line was injected into mice and three weeks later, melanomas were removed from the lungs. These cells were cultured and then injected into another mouse. Once again, melanoma cells were taken from the lungs. This process of injection into a mouse, collection of secondary melanoma cells, and injection into another mouse was repeated ten times. The tenth cell line had the property that injection of cell into a mouse produced many more lung melanomas than the cells first used. In fact, the number of secondary melanomas produced per given number of cells correlated with the number of passages through individual mice. The workers then returned to the initial cell line and developed a series of clones, each derived from a single cell. (In this sense, a clone is a collection of cells that are all descendants of a single cell.) Testing these clones by injection into mice, they showed that the cells of the primary tumor did not all have the same potential to metastasize to the lung in that some clones produced more lung melanomas than others. Thus, the primary melanoma was heterogeneous with respect to the lung-seeking ability of the individual cells, and by repeatedly collecting cells that had established themselves in the lung, increasing lung-seeking ability was selected. There is little understanding of this phenomenon at the biochemical level, but it is clear that specificity does exist for particular cell lines.

A specific surface molecule, oncofetal antigen, may be involved in targeting of mouse lymphoma to the liver, as shown by the following experiment. Cells of a specific line of mouse lymphoma were injected into a mouse. Some weeks later many secondary liver tumors formed. However, when the lymphoma cells were pretreated with an antibody directed against oncofetal antigen, which caused the cells to be coated with the antibody, liver tumors did not arise and the mice did not die. In accord with this result, in a mixing experiment lymphoma cells stuck to liver cell clusters but lymphoma cells treated with antibody did not.

SUMMARY

Cells adhere to one another in a cell-specific way. Decreasing adhesiveness is one of the most important properties of cancer cells that enable them to invade and metastasize. Metastasis occurs in the following sequence: separation of cells from the primary tumor; invasion of these cells into blood vessels, lymph vessels, or sloughing off into body cavities; transport of cancer cells via the blood and lymph systems; arrest of tumor cells in the capillaries at secondary sites; invasion of the cancer cells through the capillary walls; ingrowth of new capillaries into the tumor mass; and development of a secondary tumor. Each of these steps has a potential for control of metastasis. At present, use of anticoagulants to prevent arrest of tumor cells in a capillary clot or destruction of the factor that promotes vascularization are receiving considerable interest.

ADDITIONAL READINGS

Fidler, I.J. 1978. "Tumor heterogeneity and the biology of cancer invasion and metastasis." Canc. Res., 38, 2651.

Folkman, J. 1976. "The vascularization of tumors." Scient. Amer., 234, 58.

Maugh, T.H. 1982. "New angiogenesis inhibitor identified." Science, 216, 1304.

Nicholson, G.L. 1982. "Cell surfaces and cancer metastasis." Hospit. Pract., August, 75.

Oppenheimer, S.B. 1980. Introduction to Embryonic Development. Allyn and Bacon.

Oppenheimer, S.B. 1983. "Control of the spread of cancer." Amer. Clin. Prod. Rev., 2, 12.

Poste, G. and I.J. Fidler. 1980. "The pathogenesis of cancer metastasis." Nature, 283, 139.

Ting, C.C, S.C. Tsai, and M.J. Rogers. 1977. "Host control of tumor growth." Science 197, 571.

Willis, R.A. 1973. The Spread of Tumors in the Human Body. Butterworth.

Wood, S. 1958. "Pathogenesis of metastasis formation observed in the rabbit ear chamber." AMA Arch. Path., 66, 550.

Wood, S., E.D. Holyoke, and J.H. Yardley. 1966. "Mechanisms of metastasis production by bloodborne cancer cells." Canad. Canc. Conf., 4, 167.

6

Cancer-causing Agents: Chemicals, Radiation, and Viruses

About 85 percent of human cancers are induced by environmental agents. In this chapter we will examine three major groups of cancer-causing agents: (1) chemicals, (2) radiation, and (3) viruses. We will pay particular attention to the modes by which these agents affect cells and to possible means of preventing them from causing cellular transformation. In addition, we will see how carcinogens are identified.

CHEMICAL CARCINOGENS

A variety of different chemicals are carcinogenic. The main feature that most of these molecules have in common is that they can react with nucleic acids. Whereas a few carcinogens seem to react preferentially with proteins or RNA molecules, rather than DNA molecules, there is little doubt that most carcinogens act primarily by reaction with the bases of DNA. Those that act on RNA may cause cancer by the nongenetic mechanisms suggested in Chapter 2, for example, by altering regulatory molecules.

Many substances that are considered to be carcinogens because they cause cancer in animals are actually not carcinogenic themselves. Instead, they are fairly innocuous molecules that are changed in the body to potent carcinogens. Since the higher animals evolved, their bodies have been exposed to numerous toxic substances in the environment, some even in healthful foods. To survive the potentially deleterious effects of these substances, enzymatic systems have evolved (most are in the liver) that convert the harmful substances to harmless molecules. These enzymes constitute what is called the detoxifying system of the liver; they are contained in a component of liver cells called the microsomal fraction. However, when these enzymes encounter many fundamentally harmless manmade compounds and some fairly rare naturally occurring compounds, they convert these molecules into carcinogens. An example is the substance benzo(a)pyrene, a compound found in tobacco smoke, which is converted into a potent carcinogen by the action of enzymes called oxygenases (Figure 6-1). Sometimes, more than one enzymatic reaction may be involved in producing the ultimate carcinogen.

Since we require no knowledge of chemistry in this book, we will not go into the reactions of carcinogens with DNA. Although it is difficult to generalize, one may state that most carcinogens act in one of three ways: (1) They attack a base and change its base-pairing

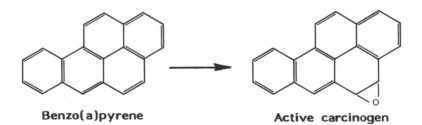

Benzo(a)pyrene   Active carcinogen

FIGURE 6-1   Activation of benzo(a)pyrene by enzymes in the liver to form an active carcinogen.

properties, resulting in a mutation in the next round of DNA replication. (2) They damage DNA in a way that temporarily blocks DNA synthesis; the response of the cell to the blockage is to set in motion an alternative pathway for DNA synthesis in which replication errors (and hence mutations) occur. (3) They insert themselves into DNA between base pairs and in a subsequent round of DNA replication cause bases to be lost or added to the sequence. The effectiveness of a carcinogen is usually related to a combination of its ability to bind to DNA (probably more than 99% of all known carcinogens act directly or indirectly on DNA) and the type of chemical alterations it produces.

A few carcinogens bind to proteins rather than to DNA. For example, dimethylnitrosamine reacts with the amino acid histidine. The manner by which carcinogens that bind to proteins cause cancer is not known at all. The most reasonable suggestion is that the binding to protein is a first step in the delivery of the carcinogen to the DNA; either the carcinogen is activated by the liver detoxifying system only when bound to the protein, or the protein-carcinogen complex can bind to DNA and thereby cause a reaction with a DNA base. These carcinogens have not been studied in detail. Other carcinogens are known that seem to react exclusively with RNA; their mode of action is also obscure.

Many carcinogens appear to be somewhat organ-specific in their effects. That is, these carcinogens cause cancers in one or a few organs, but not in other organs. Often this is the case because of the ways in which the chemicals come into contact or accumulate in certain body tissues. Probably the most obvious example is the effect of carcinogens that are breathed in, such as cigarette smoke, asbestos, nickel compounds, and chromium compounds; these cause lung cancer. Other examples are the aflatoxins, carcinogens produced by the mold Aspergillus flavus, which grows on foods such as peanuts and grains; these substances accumulate in the liver, where they are activated, and cause liver cancer. Saccharin, an artificial sweetener that passes into the urine, is suspected of producing bladder cancer. Drinking certain so-called medicinal teas appear to cause esophageal cancer. Heavy metals like arsenic, beryllium, cadmium, lead, and nickel are also associated with some specific cancers: beryllium with bone cancer and lead with kidney cancer, leukemia, and bowel cancer. The reason for the specificity with the heavy metals is not known.

In Chapter 11 on cancer epidemiology, we shall examine the question of carcinogens and specific cancers in the context of population groupings with known exposure to specific substances. In that chapter, we shall see that when groups of people are exposed to specific carcinogens in the workplace or through dietary habits, their risks of specific cancers markedly increase. These sorts of statistical correlations are very important in determining whether a given substance is carcinogenic in human beings.

INHIBITION OF THE ACTION OF CARCINOGENS

Since the environment is flooded with carcinogens, we have two approaches to protect ourselves: (1) avoidance, obviously the best solution, and (2) exposure to anticarcinogens, an "antidote" as it were. There is considerable controversy about the effectiveness of so-called anticarcinogens, though some substances in large quantities probably reduce the effectiveness of carcinogens. A few of these will be described in this section.

Several nutritional factors may help to protect individuals from the action of some carcinogens. For example, vitamin A and its analogs (retinoids) have been found to prevent cancer induced by certain carcinogens in rats. In one experiment, rats were given three biweekly doses of the carcinogen N-methyl-N-nitrosourea into the bladder. Some of these rats were then treated with either low or high doses of the vitamin A analog 13-cis-retinoic acid by addition of the retinoid to the diet for eight months. The animals were then killed, and the bladder surface was examined. The rats fed the high dose of retinoic acid had a marked reduction in the number and the size of tumors in the bladder. It should be emphasized that the retinoids did not eliminate the action of the carcinogen, but did reduce its effectiveness.

Other studies have shown that vitamin A can completely prevent lung cancers induced by some carcinogens in hamsters. The mode of action of vitamin A in these experiments has not yet been determined, but some studies suggest that binding of carcinogen to cellular DNA may be reduced. In one study, it was shown that much more of the carcinogen benzo(a)pyrene binds to the DNA of epithelial cells of the trachea taken from animals starved for vitamin A than to tracheal epithelium cells from animals with normal amounts of vitamin A in the diet. Vitamin A also stimulates specific differentiation in several cell types; since cancer cells are usually less differentiated than normal cells, it is possible that vitamin A either prevents the cells from reverting to the less differentiated cancer state or brings cancer cells back to normalcy. At present, these notions must be considered to be hypothetical. To complicate matters even more, in studies with some carcinogens vitamin A seemed to enhance effectiveness. Clearly, much is still to be learned about the relationship between vitamin A and carcinogen activity.

It has also been proposed that vitamin C may inhibit development of some cancers, and a few studies have suggested that vitamin C may increase the survival time of patients with some terminal cancers. If vitamin C does indeed exert a protective effect, it probably does so by blocking the formation of carcinogens produced in the body from precarcinogens. For example, nitrosamines (and other N-nitroso compounds) can form in the acid conditions of the stomach as a result of a reaction between the widely used food preservative sodium nitrite and specific amines. Vitamin C binds to nitrite and thereby lowers the amount of available nitrite that can combine with amine to form nitrosamines. It has been shown that animals fed both amines and sodium nitrite have a lower incidence of cancer if they are simultaneously fed vitamin C.

High levels of riboflavin (another vitamin) in the diet of rats fed carcinogenic azo dyes substantially reduced the induction of liver cancers. Azo dyes cause a rapid depletion of riboflavin in the liver, and high levels of added riboflavin counteract this effect. It is thought that riboflavin reacts with a variety of carcinogens, eliminating their carcinogenic activity.

The amount one eats and what one eats may also influence cancer rates, though a proper statistical analysis has not been carried out with human populations. This suggestion is derived from experiments that show that spontaneous mammary tumors, leukemia, and lung cancers in mice are reduced if caloric intake is restricted. Reducing food intake also decreased the incidence of skin cancer induced by dibenzanthacene. Liver cancers induced by azo dyes were reduced in animals fed with saturated fat instead of unsaturated fat. The mechanisms by which these dietary factors may reduce the induction of cancers are not understood at all.

Hormonal status also affects the susceptibility of animals to carcinogens. For example, removal of the pituitary, thyroid, or adrenal gland of rats prevented induction of liver cancer by a variety of carcinogens. If animals are given high levels of specific hormones, induction of liver cancer by some carcinogens is greatly increased. It is likely that normal hormones maintain the activity of the oxygenase enzymes (in the liver detoxification system) that activate these carcinogens. If hormone levels are reduced, oxygenase activity could decrease and carcinogen activation could be reduced. Hormones may also act by increasing cell division rates, which could make the cells more susceptible to transformation.

TESTING FOR CARCINOGENS

We have emphasized that cancer is mostly preventable and that most cancer is caused by carcinogens. Therefore, it is important to be able to identify carcinogens. The ultimate test of carcinogenicity is to determine by direct exposure whether an animal gets cancer (Figure 6-2). This procedure is time-consuming (often taking months to years), it cannot be done with humans for obvious reasons, and the analysis of results is statistical rather than direct. Furthermore, the results are often ambiguous in that a substance will produce cancer in one animal (e.g., rats) and not another (e.g., rabbits). Another type of test, which is quite straightforward, is to determine whether a substance can transform cells in culture. Usually loss of density dependence of growth or loss of anchorage dependence is the criterion used for carcinogenicity. However, this type of test will miss all substances that are converted to carcinogens by the liver detoxification system. A great breakthrough was the development of rapid tests that use bacteria; although these tests are certainly indirect, they shorten the time to two days, eliminate the need for statistical analysis, allow an enormous number of compounds to be tested in a brief period of time (weeks), and their results correlate with the most reliable animal tests. We will discuss the animal tests first.

Food additives and other compounds that humans may ingest are usually tested for carcinogenicity by administering the agents to small animals such as mice, rats, rabbits, and hamsters, and occasionally to dogs or monkeys. Although many agents cause cancer in all mammals, which lends significance to tests in mice, the number of

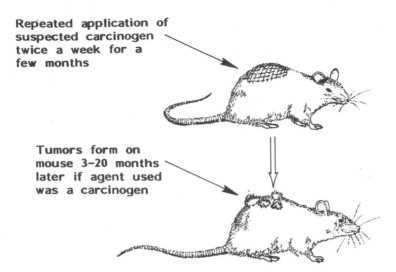

Repeated application of
suspected carcinogen
twice a week for a
few months

Tumors form on
mouse 3-20 months
later if agent used
was a carcinogen

FIGURE 6-2 A simple animal test for a carcinogen. In this case, the substance is applied to the skin. In other tests the substance may be injected or administered in food or water.

agents that appear to cause cancer in only certain mammals is sufficiently great that several different animals must be used. The differences between the animals' responses probably reflect the ways that some species metabolize inactive carcinogens. In some animals, the inactive agent may be excreted intact or modified to a harmless form, while in others the agent may be converted to an active carcinogen. However, in general, agents that cause cancer in mammals other than humans often also cause cancer in humans, so a substance that causes cancer in any animal must for the sake of public health be viewed as a human carcinogen until proved otherwise. The same considerations apply to positive results in the tests using bacteria or cultured cells.

Testing potential carcinogens on mice or rats is very expensive and takes months to years. With this in mind, new methods have been developed for initial screening of potential carcinogens. One of the most promising of these techniques measures the capacity of a substance to cause mutations in bacteria. Mutations are alterations in the DNA of the organism that are inherited by all cells descended from the mutated cell. We mentioned earlier that it is believed that many cancers are caused by DNA alterations that result in unregulated growth. If a chemical can cause mutations in bacterial DNA, such a chemical might be suspected as a possible cancer-causing agent in man. This is the rationale behind the use of bacterial tests for mutagenicity. It should be stressed that such tests are not direct assays for carcinogens; they are initial screens that provide investigators with information about which chemicals should be examined more carefully in animal test systems. Bacterial tests can be done quickly, inexpensively, and in large numbers. Therefore, they offer a way of cutting costs and time in the initial screening process.

The bacterial test, known as the Ames test, is based on the fact that most substances that test as carcinogens in animal tests are mutagens; thus, mutagenicity provides an initial screening for these hazardous agents. The Ames test uses a mutant strain of bacteria that is unable to synthesize the essential amino acid histidine (Figure 6-3). The nonmutant strain from which the mutant had been derived can grow without the addition of histidine to the medium, but these mutant bacteria will not grow in culture unless histidine is present in the medium. However, the mutation causing inability to synthesize histidine can be reversed by chemicals that cause mutations. Such a reverse mutation restores the ability to synthesize histidine, enabling the bacterium (called a revertant) once again to grow on medium lacking histidine. When a bacterium grows and divides on a solid medium, it produces a visible cluster of cells called a colony. In general, the number of colonies equals the number of bacteria put on the solid medium. However, if mutant cells that require histidine are placed on a medium lacking histidine, only about one colony will form for every 10 million cells. That is, most cells fail to multiply; the

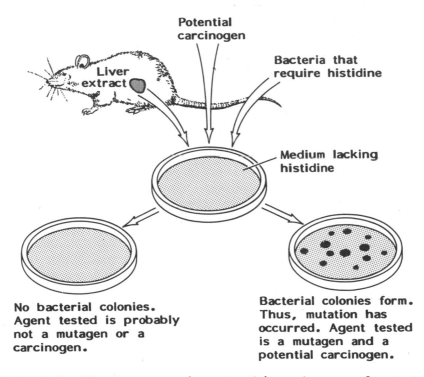

No bacterial colonies. Agent tested is probably not a mutagen or a carcinogen.

Bacterial colonies form. Thus, mutation has occurred. Agent tested is a mutagen and a potential carcinogen.

FIGURE 6-3 The Ames test for potential carcinogens. See text for details.

few colonies that form are a result of spontaneous reverse mutations from histidine deficiency (the original mutant) to histidine sufficiency (the revertant). If the mutant bacteria are exposed to a mutagen, the number of reverse mutations increases substantially, so the fraction of cells of a histidine-requiring culture that can form colonies increases. For a very effective mutagen, one colony per 100–1000 cells will form. By examining the numbers of colonies formed after treatment of the cells with a mutagen, one can get an idea of the potency of a mutagen: more colonies means that more reverse mutations have occurred. Potent mutagens are good candidates for carcinogens.

The Ames test can be performed in two ways. In the first, the mutagen is simply added to the solid medium, a known number of histidine-requiring cells are placed on the medium, and the number of colonies that form is measured. This test will indicate whether the substance is a mutagen by itself. However, recall that many substances are not carcinogenic until they are converted from harmless molecules ("precarcinogens") to carcinogens by the liver detoxification system, whose enzymes are contained in the microsomal fraction of the liver. Thus, simply by adding the microsomal fraction to the growth medium, one can test for these precarcinogens. This is the most common way to perform the Ames test. When tested in this way, about 90 percent of known carcinogens have proven to be mutagenic to bacteria and more than 90 percent of substances thought not to be carcinogenic have not caused mutations in the bacterial tests.

The Ames test has now been used with thousands of substances and mixtures (such as industrial chemicals, food additives, pesticides, hair dyes, and cosmetics), and numerous unsuspected substances have been found to stimulate reversion in this test. It is important to recognize that a high frequency of reversion does not mean that the substance is definitely a carcinogen but only that it has a high probability (about 90%) of being so. As a result of these tests, many industries have reformulated their products: for example, the cosmetic industry has changed the formulation of many hair dyes and cosmetics to render them nonmutagenic. This test has revolutionized the testing of carcinogens, because it is now practical and feasible for chemical companies and government agencies to screen all new chemicals before major investments are made in their production. Ultimately, all substances that test as mutagens must be tested further in animals, but the bacterial tests vastly rescue the number of substances that must be tested. It seems likely that the bacterial tests will be a major factor responsible for the identification and eventual reduction of carcinogens in the environment.

Animal and microbe tests do not provide the only evidence concerning whether a chemical can or cannot cause cancer, and in fact a large number of carcinogens were identified long before these tests were used. A great deal of data is available from statistical studies in which the incidence of cancer in groups with specific occupations, habits (for example, smokers), diets, and ethnic backgrounds is examined. These analyses have provided strong evidence that cigarette tar, asbestos, benzene, vinyl chloride, soot, tars, and a variety of other substances can cause cancer in humans. Significant information has come from studies of changing cancer rates among ethnic groups that have moved and changed their habits (for example, the incidence of stomach cancer is lower in Japanese Americans than among Japan still living in Japan).

The paragraphs above seem to imply that detection of carcinogens is simple, and indeed this is often the case. However, many substances still go undetected or are detected only after enormous effort. A major example is that of substances that score as negative in bacterial and cell culture tests, but cause cancer many years after a person is exposed to the agent. Statistical studies indicate that some substances may not produce cancer for 25 years or more. Other substances cause cancer only after cells have been exposed to a second agent. (Later in this chapter we will discuss the multistep aspect of cancer induction.) It may be that many potential carcinogens go undetected because the correct second agent was not used in any test. The difficulty in determining whether a substance is hazardous is illustrated by sodium nitrite, a preservative widely used in certain meat products and mentioned earlier in this chapter. Nitrite by itself is a mutagen, yet it probably does not survive the stomach acid. Nitrosamine, a product of the reaction between sodium nitrite and amine, is a potent carcinogen. For many years there has been a controversy regarding the formation of nitrosamine in the human body after ingestion of sodium nitrite. Some studies indicate that nitrosamine is formed, but in such small amounts that it is difficult to know whether what is formed in this way is hazardous. Recent studies have indicated that nitrosamine is actually formed directly when bacon, which contains sodium nitrite, is cooked (most meats preserved with nitrites are eaten cold). As a result of these new findings, federal regulatory agencies are presently working on stringent guidelines for the use of sodium nitrite in bacon and any meat products that are heated at high temperatures. One may argue that just to be sure, nitrite should not be used as a preservative. However, an argument can be made to counter this suggestion. When meat is stored, it often becomes contaminated with microscopic amounts of fungi. One of these fungi makes aflatoxin, a potent carcinogen. Thus, eliminating one potential hazard may introduce another real hazard. Of course, one solution is to eliminate all stored meats from the diet (thereby eliminating two potential carcinogens), but as we pointed out in the beginning of the book, changing the eating habits of a population is not a simple thing to do. In general, decisions to regulate hazardous substances are difficult and are often based on economic considerations and habit, as well as health-related factors. The awareness by the public of the danger of potential carcinogens in the environment is increasing, and such awareness should bring added pressure on those responsible for protecting the people from environmental carcinogens and should help individuals themselves to choose habits that may reduce cancer risk. What we are saying is that at present in many cases the only thing that the government can do is to provide information and leaves choices and decisions to the individual.

RADIATION CARCINOGENESIS

Radiation can cause cancer. Both particulate radiations, such as neutrons, electrons, and alpha particles, and electromagnetic radiation, such as ultraviolet light and x rays, have been shown to cause cancer or cell transformation in numerous animals and experimental systems. In addition, good evidence has accumulated that many human cancers have been caused by radiation. The most striking example is the large number of cases of leukemia and other cancers that appeared in the populations of Hiroshima and Nagasaki in Japan many years after the atom bomb blasts. Detailed analysis of the doses received by individuals (measured by their known distance from the explosion) and the leukemia frequency has shown that there is a strict correlation between cancer incidence and dose received.

Evidence other than bomb data also indicates clearly that radiation can cause cancer in humans. Most of the data comes from populations that have inadvertently been exposed to various radiations. For example, the incidence of thyroid cancer is elevated in individuals who have been treated for various reasons with radioactive iodine (which accumulates in the thyroid). Ringworm of the scalp was once treated by x irradiation of the head in the children; a significant number of these children developed cancer in the head and neck 10-20 years later. Bone cancer is common in individuals who early in the century used radium to paint fluorescent dials of watches; radium is chemically related to calcium and hence accumulates in bone. A variety of cancers, especially skin cancer, occur to a great extent in individuals who had jobs that exposed them to x rays and radioactive chemicals or who worked either on the atom bomb or in the nuclear industry. Skin cancer is also more prevalent in the sun belts of the United States, especially among fair-skinned people and individuals who work outdoors.

The fact that ionizing radiation causes cancer raises important questions about the use of x rays in diagnosis. There is no doubt that the use of diagnostic x rays has saved many lives, but the risk of cancer induction by these tests must be kept in mind. These considerations have had two consequences: (1) ultrasensitive x-ray films have been developed that enable much smaller doses of radiation to be used, and (2) routine and massive x-ray screening is not carried out without reason. For example, the use of x rays to detect breast lumps that may be cancerous has decreased in the younger age groups. Women are no longer given routine mammography and xeroradiography unless they are in specific risk categories in which the benefit is believed to outweigh the potential risk. That is, for these tests to be useful the number of breast cancers detected early enough for cure must exceed by a wide margin the number of breast cancers that may be induced by the radiation. Statistical analysis indicates that if all women, independent of their risk group, were routinely irradiated at regular times, the number induced would be greater than the number detected. Hopefully, new technology yielding a substantial reduction of the required dose could change the ratio of benefit to risk.

The kind of damage produced by radiation has been well documented. There is no doubt that the major damage is to DNA, and indeed radiation increases mutation frequency considerably. There are basically three kinds of damage that occur: breaks in the individual single strands of DNA, double-strand breaks in which the whole DNA molecule is fragmented, and alteration of bases. Single-strand breaks are efficiently repaired. Double-strand breaks cause cell death, but can also be repaired, occasionally with the result that different chromosomes exchange fragments (translocation). As will be seen in Chapter 8, such exchange may lead to activation of oncogenes (genes that cause cancer). It is likely that base damage, which is highly mutagenic, is the major cause of radiation-induced cancer. X rays and gamma rays are also used to treat a variety of cancers, as will be discussed in Chapter 13. Double-strand breakage is probably the major cause of the killing of cancer cells in these treatments.

The relations between radiation and mutation mentioned above is not the only explanation of radiation-induced carcinogenesis. In some experimental systems, radiation probably causes cancer by activating certain leukemia viruses already present in a latent state in the animals. How the activation occurs is not known, but it probably is a side effect of the repair of radiation damage to DNA elsewhere in the cell.

STEPS IN CARCINOGENESIS

That the induction of cancer is a multistage process was first proposed more than sixty years ago from studies of virus-induced tumors and from the cocarcinogenic effect of a plant extract called croton oil. The initial observation was made by Peyton Rous, who found that certain virus-induced tumors (papillomas) in rabbits often regressed (became smaller and ultimately disappeared) after a fairly short period of time. However, the papillomas could be made to reappear if the skin was stressed by punching small holes in it or by the application of irritating substances. He proposed that tumor cells could remain in a dormant state from which they could be activated. The first step in conversion of a normal cell to a latent tumor cell was called initiation. The second step, in which the tumor cells were triggered to grow without control was called promotion. Later experiments confirmed this conclusion. In these experiments it was shown that if the skin of mice was painted once with the carcinogen methylcholanthrene, only a small number of animals developed tumors. However, if at a later time the same area was painted repeatedly (weekly) with croton oil, which is not by itself carcinogenic, the animals developed skin cancers. In the course of the next 20 years it became clear that some substances were initiators and others were only promoters.

Continued study of this phenomenon has made it fairly clear that initiation, which requires only a single and short application of the initiator, is a permanent change that is inherited by progeny cells. Thus, it seems clear that in most cases initiation is a mutational event. This agrees with the fact that almost all initiators test as mutagens in the Ames and other tests, and many bind directly to DNA. (Other proof will be given in Chapter 8 when oncogenes are are described.) Promotion, the second step in cancer induction, seems to be an event in which initiated cells (that is, latent tumor cells) are stimulated to divide and to express altered genetic information. This agrees with the fact that mitogens (substances or agents that stimulate mitosis) are promoters and that repeated tissue injury and irritation, which usually causes repair and cell division, causes cancer. A striking example of the role of cell division can be seen in the promotion of liver cancer induced by radiation. Application of small doses of x rays to rats produces a particular number of liver tumors. However, if (perhaps many months later) a portion of the liver is surgically excised, the liver begins to regenerate and numerous tumors form. Without the previous x radiation excision of part of the liver does not cause liver cancer.

It is important to recognize that initiation and promotion must both occur and that they must occur in the right sequence. That is, application of a promoter before an initiator will not lead to cancer. Furthermore, the promoter can be applied months or even a year after the application of the initiator, and a cancer still forms.

It is likely that most, if not all, cancers in man may result from a two-step process. This is suggested by the fact that most tumors require a very long time to develop. For example, many precancerous conditions (for example, chronic sores, moles) are known in humans that remain static for 10-20 years and then become malignant. Cervical carcinoma often begins as a localized nonspreading condition characterized by abnormal cell types. This precancerous condition may become a malignant spreading cancer several years later. Also, as we have mentioned repeatedly, exposure to a carcinogen often does not result in a cancer until many years later. Presumably. the precancerous state is achieved by initiation, while the malignancy develops only after promotion has occurred. A few examples are known in which infection of some animals by certain viruses causes rapid development of tumors. These viruses contain genes that provide both the initiation and promotion events.

Let us expand on the essential features of initiation and promotion, for understanding them provides a useful way to think about cancer prevention. Initiation can occur after a single, brief exposure to a carcinogen. From the length of the exposure it is clear that conversion of a normal cell to a latent tumor cell can occur within one mitotic cycle. In addition, initiation is irreversible. Finally, the change is likely to be a genetic one (that is, a mutation), since the ability to become a tumor cell is inherited by all progeny of the cell originally exposed to the initiator. (It is possible though to produce a nongenetic change in expression of a gene that is carried through from generation to generation.) In contrast with initiation, the promotion phase is a slow gradual process, requiring long exposure to the promoting agent. It may be that promotion is a single but highly improbable event, which would account for the repeated exposure that is needed for promotion to be consummated. Promotion is reversible, since it can sometimes be reversed by application of anticarcinogens some time after exposure to the promoter. The complete process of promotion can be thought of as occurring also in two stages. In the first, an initiated cell multiplies and produces a small clone of latent tumor cells (which might be recognized as a precancerous cluster of cells). The second stage is called tumor progression, in which altered cells multiply and continue to change somewhat, losing growth control and escaping from various (unknown) defense mechanisms of the host.

Note that the tumor is not necessarily malignant; it may remain benign indefinitely or at a later time lose adhesiveness (anchorage dependence?) and begin to slough off cells and metastasize.

One of the best-studied classes of promoters are the phorbol esters (components of croton oil, the first promoter detected). These substances cause a wide variety of biochemical effects on cultured cells. Of some interest, these effects are quite like those produced by epidermal growth factor (Chapter 4), a point that should be remembered when we discuss oncogenes in Chapter 8.

The concept of initiation and promotion can be applied to the inherited cancers. We mentioned in an earlier chapter that some cancers, for example, bilateral retinoblastoma, are inherited as a single gene. All people carrying the gene develop the cancer, but time is required and the number of tumors is small, even though every cell in the body carries the gene. The fact that there is only a single location of the tumor can be explained by assuming that the gene can be expressed and that the tumor cells can only grow in certain environments. However, the delay of many years before the tumor appears and the small number of tumors certainly reflects the low probability of promotion. That is, because the retinoblastoma gene is already present, initiation is unnecessary, but the slow process, promotion, is still required.

The fact that initiation is a very brief event and promotion requires a lengthy exposure has profound implications for cancer prevention. For example, it seems that if promoters could be eliminated from our environment, human cancer might be avoided. Such an approach is more feasible than eliminating initiators, since exposure to them can be very short and is irreversible. However, since promotion may require 10-20 years, even reducing the number or concentration of promoters in the environment by a factor of 10 might increase the time required for promotion to 40-50 years. This would mean a normal life expectancy for most individuals, in that death would normally come from other causes before cancer ever developed.

IRRITATION AND CANCER

In the preceding section we noted that irritation might be the promotion step in some cancers. The idea that chronic physical irritation can promote development of cancer is an old one, but only recently have experimental results supported the notion. In one set of experiments rats were inoculated with a single dose of the carcinogen N-nitroso-N-methylurea, which by itself produces tumors at almost any site in the body. These rats were also subjected to constant irritation of an area in the mouth by a stainless steel wire wrapped around a tooth and projecting onto the check lining. More malignant tumors were found in the area irritated by the wire than in any other area of the body of the rats treated with the carcinogen. No tumors were observed in rats with the wire but not given the carcinogen, or in rats with neither the wire nor the carcinogen. Some workers have suggested that the effects of a carcinogen need not be exerted on cells that eventually will become transformed into cancer cells. Instead, the carcinogen may cause a loss or reduction of the ability of an organ such as the liver to secrete substances that prevent multiplication of some cell types. Tumors could then appear at locations where the proliferative capacity of cells is increased by normal physiological processes or by long-term irritation (for example, by the wire) or by wounding. The experiment just described has been taken as support for this contention. The interpretation is based on some data that suggest that the carcinogen used acts primarily on the liver.

VIRAL CARCINOGENESIS

Many viruses are known that cause cancer. The first cancer virus detected was the Rous sarcoma virus. It was first extracted from chicken tumors; when inoculated into tumor-free birds, tumors formed shortly afterward (Figure 6-4). This process can also be seen in culture by infecting normal chicken cells with the virus; in a few days they develop growth habits characteristic of tumor cells, namely, lack of contact inhibition of growth and movement of the cells, and other properties described in Chapter 4. Furthermore, the transformed cells form tumors when inoculated into young chickens.

The mechanism by which most viruses cause tumors will be presented in Chapter 8, where we discuss oncogenes. At this point we will only present some of the evidence for cancer induction by viruses in humans.

In early experiments the test of a virus as a causative agent of cancer was to show that cancer can be transmitted to a healthy animal by injection with an extract of tumor tissue. However, in many cases this test fails, for the viruses will not establish themselves in the healthy animal, being destroyed by the animal's immune system. This difficulty can often be circumvented by injecting newborn animals. This latter technique was used in an important experiment that showed that mouse leukemia was caused by a virus. It had been observed that the mouse strain C58 had a very high incidence of "spontaneous" leukemia, whereas strain CH3 mice rarely developed the disease. Injection of CH3 mice with extracts of leukemic cells from C58 failed to produce leukemia, but if newborn CH3 mice were injected with the extract, the incidence of leukemia went up dramatically. Some of the mice did not get leukemia, but their offspring had an incidence of leukemia as high as the strain C58 mice. Thus, this experiment showed that not only could a cancer-causing agent be transmitted from one mouse to another by a virus, but also that the propensity to get leukemia was carried from generation to generation. Many years later it was shown that the virus DNA becomes incorporated into the mouse chromosomes, so viral genes are inherited as mouse genes. The presence of the viral genes bypasses the need for initiation and later in the life of a carrier animal, expression of the viral genes is triggered by exposure to chemicals, radiation, irritation, etc. (that is, a promoter of some kind), the virus becomes active, and leukemia develops. Since these early experiments hundreds of tumor viruses have been isolated that can cause cancer when infecting a newborn and that can be inherited. An important feature of many of these viruses, which has not yet been explained, is that a particular virus

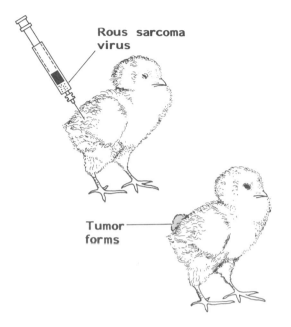

FIGURE 6-4 Development of cancer in a chick several weeks to months after inoculation with Rous sarcoma virus.

may cause cancer in one host and an infectious disease in another. For example, the virus SV40, which causes harmless infections in monkeys, induces sarcomas and leukemia in newborn hamsters; and adenoviruses, which cause the common cold in humans, induces sarcomas when injected into newborn rats and hamsters.

For many of the animal viruses the viral infection is transmitted from one animal to the next. For instance, leukemias and lymphomas caused by feline leukemia virus can be transmitted between cats living in close proximity. Transmission usually occurs when the animals are quite young. Furthermore, even when there is no evidence for infectivity of certain cancers, nonetheless the great majority of animal cancers seem to involve a virus. Fortunately, a good deal of evidence shows that there is no transmission of this virus from cats or other animals to humans.

The situation with humans seems to be quite different. Before describing the role of viruses in human cancer, one must understand how a cancer virus would be identified in a human, since clearly one cannot test potential cancer viruses by injecting them into humans. We consider first a cancer called Burkitt's lymphoma. The initial suspicion that this cancer was caused by an infectious agent was based on the observation that the disease was found only in a well-defined region of equatorial East Africa. Cells cultured from the tumors were found to contain a virus now known as Epstein-Barr (EB) virus. Since then, much circumstantial evidence has accumulated that suggests that the virus is the cause of the lymphoma: (1) patients with the cancer have a high concentration of antibodies directed against the virus compared to individuals that do not have the cancer, suggesting that the patients have had substantial infections with the virus; (2) the tumor cells all contain one copy of viral DNA linearly integrated into one of the chromosomes (integration of viral DNA is discussed further in Chapter 8); (3) EB virus transforms normal human cells in culture; and (4) the virus induces cancer when injected into certain monkeys and apes. The evidence is substantial for the virus as an agent of the cancer, but nonetheless it cannot be the sole cause of the cancer. The virus occurs throughout the world, yet the cancer is restricted to parts of Africa and New Guinea having the same climate. Furthermore, the virus is identical to the one that causes infectious mononucleosis in Caucasians in North America, so clearly other factors, as yet unknown, are involved. Another cancer associated with EB virus is cancer of the nasopharynx; here the circumstantial evidence is the same as that given above for Burkitt's lymphoma.

Epidemiological data for cancer of the cervix also suggests that a virus might be involved. The prime evidence is that cervical cancer is associated with early sexual activity and having a large number of sexual partners. A herpes virus, HSV-2, is suspected, primarily because women with invasive cervical cancer usually have higher concentrations of antibody to the virus than women without the cancer. Hepatitis B virus is thought to be associated with certain liver cancers (primary hepatocellular carcinoma). The evidence, which is again circumstantial, is the following: (1) the disease occurs most frequently in certain regions of Asia and Africa in which hepatitis is common, (2) patients with the particular cancer generally have high concentrations of antibody to the virus in their blood, suggesting an early and prolonged infection, and (3) individuals who have had hepatitis have a higher probability of developing the cancer than people who never had hepatitis. Recently, a vaccine has been developed to prevent hepatitis caused by the virus, and it is currently being used in Asia and Africa. If the incidence of primary hepatocellular carcinoma decreases in the coming years among the vaccinated population, the connection between the virus and cancer will be established.

Of recent interest is the disease AIDS (acquired immunity deficiency syndrome). Patients with AIDS frequently develop a highly malignant skin cancer called Kaposi's sarcoma. AIDS has definitely been found to be caused by a particular virus, human T-cell leukemia virus III.

When considering viruses as a cause of human cancer, the question of whether one can catch cancer immediately arises. In fact, there is no evidence whatsoever that cancer can be acquired by direct infection. A virus infection can certainly be transmitted, but clearly the virus itself is insufficient to cause cancer. For example, EB virus, which can cause cancer, normally does not; in fact, it is carried by a large fraction of the population of North America and Europe. Most humans harbor herpes virus, yet only a small fraction have cancers associated with herpes virus. Even in the case of AIDS, which is clearly a viral disease that is transmitted, all AIDS patients do not develop Kaposi's sarcoma, often a cause of death among AIDS patients. Obviously, other factors are necessary for cancers to develop. In fact, it is generally believed that most human cancers are caused by chemical carcinogens and radiation and that viral infection only provides the initiation step (that is, induces a predisposition to develop cancer). Most of the known tumor viruses in animals contain RNA rather than DNA as their genetic material. To date, only one RNA virus, human T-cell leukemia virus, has been isolated that is associated with human cancer. We will have much more to say about how viruses cause cancer in Chapter 8, where oncogenes carried by viruses are described.

SUMMARY

The major types of agents that cause cancer are chemicals, radiation, and viruses. Most of these agents appear to exert their effects at the level of the gene. New, rapid tests designed to detect the mutagenic potential of various suspect agents offer hope that many more of these agents will be identified as potential carcinogens and eliminated from our environment. Study of the mode of action of carcinogens is leading both to a better understanding of cancer causation and to a means of preventing carcinogen-induced cell transformation.

ADDITIONAL READINGS

Ames, B.W., Durston, W.E., Hamasaki, E., and Lee, F.D. 1973. "Carcinogens are mutagens: A simple test system combining liver homogenates for activation and bacteria for detection." Proc. Natl. Acad. Sci. USA, 70, 2281.

Ames, B.W. 1979. "Identifying environmental chemicals causing mutations and cancer." Science, 204. 587.

Baltimore, D. 1976. "Viruses, polymerases and cancer." Science, 192, 632.

Berenblum, I. 1974. Carcinogenesis as a Biological Problem. Elsevier-North Holland.

Cole, L.J., and Nowell, P.C. 1965. "Radiation carcinogenesis: the sequence of events." Science, 150, 1782.

Enomoto, M., and Saito, M. 1972. "Carcinogens produced by fungi." Ann. Rev. Microbiol., 26, 279.

Epstein, S.S. 1974. "Environmental determinants of human cancer." Cancer Res., 32, 2425.

Gross, L. 1970. Oncogenic Viruses. Pergamon.

Hiatt, H.H., J.D. Watson, and J.A. Winsten. 1977. <u>Origins of Human Cancer</u>. Cold Spring Harbor.

Huberman, E., R. Mager, and L. Sachs. 1976. "Mutagenesis and transformation of normal cells by chemical carcinogens." <u>Nature</u>, 264, 360.

Miller, E.C. 1978. "Some current perspectives on chemical carcinogens in humans and experimental animals." <u>Cancer Res</u>., 38, 1479.

Miller, J. A. 1970. "Carcinogenesis by chemicals: An overview." <u>Cancer Res</u>., 30, 559.

Miller, R. W. 1972. "Radiation-induced cancer." <u>J. Natl. Cancer Inst.</u>, 49, 1221.

Rous, P. 1911. "A sarcoma of fowl transmissible by an agent separable from tumor cells." <u>J. Expt. Med.</u>, 13, 397.

Ruddon, R.W. 1981. <u>Cancer Biology</u>. Oxford.

Ryser, H.. 1971. "Chemical carcinogenesis." <u>New Eng. J. Med.</u>, 285, 721.

Setlow, R. B. 1978. "Repair-deficient human disorders and cancer." <u>Nature</u>, 271, 713.

Weisburger, J.H., and Weisburger, E.K. 1966. "Chemicals as causes of cancer." <u>Chem. Eng. News</u>, 43, 124-142.

7

Genetics of Cancer

In this chapter, we will examine (1) evidence that some cancers are inherited according to specific genetic principles, (2) evidence that some cancers are caused by an interplay of specific genes and environmental agents, and (3) experiments that have led to the identification of specific chromosomes involved in transformation of human cells into cancer cells.

Some cancers can be inherited, and others are often associated with specific chromosomal aberrations. Recall from Chapter 3 that a large number of patients with chronic myeloid leukemia have a chromosomal abnormality in which the long arm of chromosome 22 is shortened as a result of a piece of this arm being translocated, usually to the end of the long arm of chromosome 9. In addition, individuals with this chromosomal abnormality, but who are free of leukemia, almost always develop the disease at a later time. Individuals with three, rather than the normal two, copies of certain chromosomes (such as chromosome 21) have increased incidence of leukemia. Patients with meningioma (cancer of the membranes around nerves) usually lack either a chromosome 22 or chromosome 8, and patients with Burkitt's lymphoma usually have an alteration of chromosome 14. Furthermore, in an extensive survey of thousands of cancer patients all cancer cells examined had an abnormal chromosome number. Other studies have shown that as a cell line that has been transformed in culture is carried through many generations, increasing numbers of chromosomal abnormalities are observed. Accompanying this change is increasing malignancy; that is, if the cultured cells are transplanted into an animal, those with greater numbers of chromosomes produce tumors with a greater degree of invasiveness, as determined by the number of different locations of tumors.

Chromosomal abnormalities are associated with cancer in two different ways. In one case only the cancer cells possess the abnormality, so one can probably conclude that the abnormality developed either during or after the transformation from normal to cancer cell. However, in some cancer patients all cells in the body contain the abnormality; in this case, the abnormality must be inherited, and one can assume that the abnormality is either a cause of the cancer, a prerequisite for cancer induction, or something that predisposes the individual to developing the cancer. Because of the multistep nature of transformation, the third possibility is probably the nearest to the truth.

INHERITED CANCERS

We have stated several times in earlier chapters that some cancers are inherited. Examination of genetic data indicates that there are several modes of inheritance of cancer. For example, some cancers are inherited by transmission of a single altered gene, which is a mode of inheritance that can be demonstrated quite easily. Others are inherited in a more complex way. Still others give hints that they are inherited, but the evidence is not always strong. We will begin this chapter with showing how a decision is made about the genetic basis of a particular cancer; then, various modes of inheritance will be described.

Pedigree Analysis as a Means of Identifying an Inherited Cancer

With animals genetic questions are usually answered by carrying out matings between animals with particular traits. Measurement of frequencies of appearance of different traits among the offspring provides the crucial information, and strong conclusions can usually be made about the genetics of the trait. If after a set of matings is performed, the information is insufficient, more matings can be carried out to provide the critical data. Obviously, with humans such experiments cannot be done. Instead, family histories (<u>pedigrees</u>) showing which individuals exhibit the trait in question provide the necessary information. An example of one such pedigree for a family with a particular cancer is shown in Figure 7-1. A hatched box or circle indicates a person with the disease. A square box is male and a circle is female.

The first thing to notice is that the cancer is present in several generations, which suggests, but does not prove, that it is inherited. Simple logic, based on principles established by Mendel, is applied to the pedigree. As a start, one assumes that a single gene determines the trait and then examines the consequences of the assumption. We shall do that and also first consider what would be expected if the trait is <u>recessive</u>. A trait is recessive if a person carrying one good

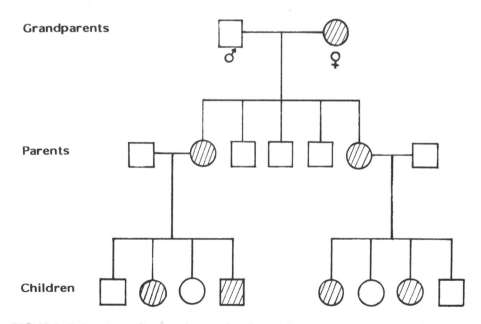

FIGURE 7-1 A pedigree for a family with numerous cases of cancer that shows that the cancer is probably determined by a dominant gene that is not carried on the X chromosome. A shaded symbol indicates that the person developed the particular cancer. Squares and circles designate males and females, respectively.

gene and one defective gene does not exhibit the trait; that is, only with two defective copies will the trait be evident. (If the trait does appear when a single defective gene is present, the trait is <u>dominant</u>.) Thus, in this pedigree, if the trait were recessive, the grandmother, who has the cancer, would have to have two copies of the defective gene. All of her eggs would have a copy of the defective gene, so all of the progeny in the second (parent) generation would carry the defective gene. Since the disease appears in the parental generation (and those having the disease must have two copies of the defective gene), the grandfather would also necessarily be a contributor of the gene to the progeny. Since the third generation progeny (children) also exhibit the cancer, the two males that married into the parental generation would also have to carry the gene. In other words, if the gene was a recessive, every parent in all three generations would have to be a carrier of the defect. Since cancers of this type are rare, it is exceedingly unlikely that so many carriers of the defect would just happen to come together and mate. Thus, we have good reason to reject the hypothesis that the gene is a recessive, so we turn to the possibility that the cancer is a dominant trait (one defective gene is sufficient to cause the cancer). This situation is diagrammed in Figure 7-2. Here we assume that the grandmother has one copy of the defective gene. Therefore, half of her eggs would carry the defective gene, and half would carry the normal gene. The grandfather, who lacks the cancer, must have two good genes, so all of his sperm carry normal genes. Therefore, half of the offspring in the second generation would get the defective gene, and, if the gene is dominant, would develop the cancer, which is observed. Following through this line of reasoning to the next generation, we note that each of the people in the second generation with the disease would have a good gene (from the grandfather) and a bad gene (from the grandmother). Thus, if each affected person in the second generation had normal mates (two good genes), only about one half of their children would also be expected to get the cancer, as observed. The data are clearly consistent with the idea that the cancer is carried by a single dominant gene.

In many cases, combined genetic analysis and microscopic examination of chromosomes can locate defects on a particular chromosome. However, by an especially simple genetic test it is possible to determine whether a gene is carried on the female X chromosome. In this pedigree we can conclude quite easily that the defective gene is not carried on the sex chromosomes. Since a male contains one X and one Y chromosome, the grandfather would have only one good gene, on his single X. Thus, if the gene were recessive, all male offspring in the second generation (they receive an X from the grandmother and a Y from the grandfather) would have the disease. If the gene were dominant, at least one of the male offspring in the second generation should have the disease. Since the cancer does not appear among the three males in the second generation, the gene is unlikely to be located on the X chromosome.

Usually, analysis of a single pedigree is not sufficient to draw an unambiguous conclusion, because the number of individuals in a given generation may not be large enough. For example, if the second

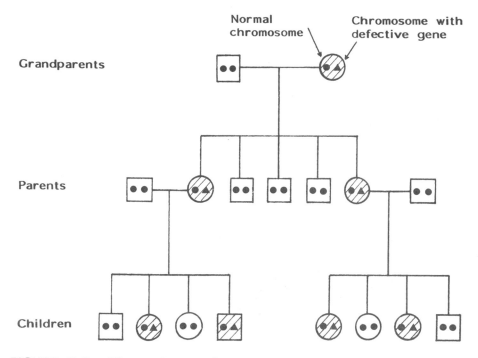

FIGURE 7-2 The pedigree shown in Figure 7-1, with the genetic constitution of each individual shown.

generation of this pedigree had no male offspring, or only one male offspring (neither of which would be particularly unusual in a human family), no statement could be made about the X chromosome. Analyses of several different families will usually provides the necessary information. In isolated cases one might argue that familial clustering of certain cancers could be caused by exposure of most or all family members to specific carcinogens. Again such an argument could hold for an isolated case, but when many pedigrees show the same pattern of inheritance, one can say with assurance that a particular cancer is inherited.

Pedigree analysis of many familial groups has shown that several cancers are inherited. Some of these cancers are described in the next section.

Cancers Inherited as a Single Dominant Gene

Retinoblastoma, which affects the retina of one or both eyes, frequently in children, is a hereditary tumor. All cases of retinoblastoma that occur in both eyes (bilateral) are inherited as a ~~dominant~~ trait not carried on the sex chromosome (in fact, the pedigree in Figure 7-1 is for a family with bilateral retinoblastoma). The disease is a rare one, occurring in about one in 20,000 children. If diagnosed

Recessive

early, death can be prevented by removal of the eyes. Patients with this disease are also more susceptible to other cancers such as leukemia and cancer of bone, kidney, and muscle.

Another disease that is inherited is familial multiple polyposis of the colon. It is inherited as a dominant trait in humans, as with retinoblastoma. Individuals with this condition develop many polyps (small well-localized growths) on the inner lining of the colon. This condition appears early in life (often before age 10). The polyps are benign (not malignant), but often become malignant. The chance of malignancy increases with increasing age of the individual with the polyposis condition.

Following is a list of other diseases inherited as dominants. Discussion of these conditions is beyond the scope of this book, but can be found in numerous medical texts.

Carotid body tumors
Cerebelloretinal hemangioblastomatosis
Familial gastrointestinal polyposis
Hereditary exostosis
Hereditary polyendocrine adenomatosis
Intraocular melanoma
Medullary thyroid carcinoma, bilateral
Multiple polyposis coli (Gardner's syndrome)
Neurofibromatosis (von Recklinghausen's disease)
Nevoid basal cell carcinoma syndrome
Phaeochromocytoma
Tuberous sclerosis
Tylosis with esophageal cancer

Cancers Inherited as a Recessive Gene

A variety of genetic diseases inherited as a recessive are associated with the predisposition to develop cancer. As pointed out in the pedigree analysis given earlier, because two copies of the defective gene are needed for the disease to be expressed, both parents must be carriers of the gene. Since the gene frequency is fairly low, the diseases are quite rare. However, within a single family there may be many carriers, so the diseases often appear in communities in which distant relatives frequently marry (inbred communities).

One of the more common disorders of this type is xeroderma pigmentosum. The cells of people with this disease are unable or less able to repair DNA that has been damaged by ultraviolet radiation. Unless the individuals rigorously avoid exposure to sunlight, they develop multiple skin cancers. Here, we see how a specific inherited condition coupled with a specific environmental agent (ultraviolet light) together lead to cancer. It is likely that many cancers result from such an interplay of genetic predisposition and environmental agents.

Bloom's syndrome, Fanconi's anemia, and ataxia telangiectasis are also recessive disorders that predispose individuals to a variety of cancers. Cells taken from individuals with these disorders display unusual chromosomal fragility in which chromosomal breakage and rearrangements occur. Such chromosomal alterations could lead to defective gene products that cause cell transformation or to altered concentrations of critical gene products that regulate cell division. These disorders are being actively studied.

A few other recessive disorders that are often associated with cancer are the following: decreased pigmentation with photophobia, dermatitis with thrombocytopenic purpura (Wiskott-Aldrich syndrome), and nystagmus with leukocytic inclusions (Chediak-Higashi syndrome).

POSSIBLE COMPLEX INHERITANCE FACTORS IN SOME CANCERS

Many cancers that do not appear by pedigree analysis to be inherited as one-gene traits nonetheless exhibit a tendency to occur in families. For example, patients with bilateral breast cancer often have had relatives with breast cancer. Individuals who smoke cigarettes and have a close relative with lung cancer have a greater risk of developing lung cancer than smokers in general. People with endometrial carcinoma (a type of uterine cancer) and certain leukemias often have relatives affected with the disease.

It is difficult to draw unambiguous conclusions about the nature of the familial distribution of these cancers, for there are three quite different possibilities: (1) the disease may result from common exposure to environmental agents or to viruses that are passed among the members of the family; (2) the disease may be determined by several genes carried on different chromosomes, which would give rise to a complex pattern inheritance that would never become evident from examination of small pedigrees; and (3) the disease is inherited as a single gene, but the expression of the gene is determined by a wide variety of factors, resulting in a lack of expression of many carriers of the gene. Only very comprehensive studies will be able to distinguish these possibilities.

There is one experimental system in which one must interpret apparent inherited cancers with caution, namely, cancer that is prevalent in clones of animals. For example, many highly inbred strains of animals have been developed for a variety of experimental purposes. It is sometimes found that certain inbred strains are exceedingly susceptible to certain cancers. For example, more than 95 percent of breeding female mice of the strain C3H develop mammary carcinomas. This seems like a clear example of a genetically determined cancer. However, such a conclusion cannot be drawn because cancer-causing viruses might be efficiently transmitted in these mouse strains, perhaps even through germ cells. Only careful genetic tests involving crosses with animals that do not develop the cancer can show whether the disease has a strict genetic basis.

INHERITANCE AND TWO-STEP MODELS OF CANCER

Inheritance of a cancer seems at first sight to preclude the notion of a requirement for two steps in cancer induction. However, the existence of both inherited and noninherited cancers is consistent with this idea. We need only recall the distinction between the irreversible initiation step and the later promotion step. In that model, a cancer is inherited if the mutation that corresponds to initiation is inherited.

If given sufficient time, the promotion step will inevitably occur, and the cancer will clearly appear to be inherited. A noninherited cancer is then one in which the first mutation (the initiation step) occurs after fertilization has occurred.

A clear example of an inherited cancer that is consistent with a two-step model of cancer induction is bilateral retinoblastoma, discussed above. Even though every cell in the body of these patients carries the retinoblastoma gene, the cancer always originates in the eye, and usually only a single tumor develops. That is, of the billions of cells in the retina, only one becomes cancerous. Thus, the presence of the retinoblastoma gene does not demand that a cell becomes cancerous, for it probably mediates only the first step; the other step must occur only very infrequently, and the probability of its occurrence is affected by the environment of the cells.

SPECIFIC HUMAN CHROMOSOMES INVOLVED IN MALIGNANT TRANSFORMATION

An elegant technique can be used to identify a human chromosome that carries a gene involved in transformation. This technique was developed originally to locate integrated tumor viral DNA. We will describe it briefly.

The technique utilizes fusion of human cells with cells of other animals in a similar way as the experiments conducted by Frye and Edidin that were described in Chapter 2. When human cells are fused with other cells, many human chromosomes are lost or ejected from the hybrid cells. By testing the hybrid (fused) cells for specific biochemical characteristics, one can determine which specific human chromosomes are lost or retained in the hybrid. In the first experiments used to map cancer genes human cells were first transformed into cancer cells with SV40 virus. These cells were fused with normal mouse cells. It was found that hybrid cells that retained the transformed properties and SV40 T antigen contained human chromosome number 7. Cells without this chromosome did not possess T antigen and were not transformed. Thus, the SV40 DNA must have been located in human chromosome 7 in the original transformed human cells. Studies with a variety of transformed cell lines showed that several locations were possible for SV40 DNA. Similar experiments have been carried out with other viruses and with the cancer genes known as oncogenes, which are described in Chapter 8.

ADDITIONAL READINGS

Croce, C. M., and Koprowski, H. 1978. "The genetics of human cancer." Scient. Amer., 238, 117.

German, J., ed. 1974. Chromosomes and Cancer. Wiley.

Heston, W. E. 1965. "Genetic factors in the etiology of cancer." Cancer Res., 25, 1320.

Mitelman, F., and L. Goran. 1976. "Clustering of aberrations to specific chromosomes in human neoplasms. II: A survey of 287 neoplasms." Hereditas, 82, 167.

Mulvihill, J.J., R.W. Miller, and J.F. Fravmeni,, eds. 1977. Genetics of Human Cancer. Raven.

Robbins, J. H., K.H. Kraemer, M.A. Letzner, B.W. Festoff, and H.G. Coon. 1974. "Xeroderma pigmentosum. An inherited disease with sun sensitivity, multiple cutaneous neoplasms and abnormal DNA repair." Ann. Intern. Med., 80, 221.

8

Oncogenes

Up to this point in this book, we have described in some detail the properties of cancer cells isolated from patients and of cells transformed in the laboratory. We have also examined a wide variety of substances and agents that cause cancer. In Chapter 3 we considered in a very general way what might cause cancer. Until the late 1970s it would not have been possible to discuss the cancer problem in any other terms, because little or nothing was known about the molecular basis of cancer. This was frustrating to most cancer researchers, since development of new treatments had to rely totally on trial and error rather than on a logical approach based on biochemical principles. The situation began to change in the early 1960s with the discovery of numerous tumor viruses and a fairly good understanding of the life cycles of these viruses. However, how a virus could cause cancer remained hypothetical, though the framework for thinking about it had been developed by Howard Temin in his provirus hypothesis. Temin recognized that when a cell was transformed by a virus to the cancerous state, its progeny, arising by repeated cell division, retained the ability to grow as a cancer. Thus, Temin proposed that a viral gene was incorporated into the cell's chromosome set, so that it could be carried through subsequent generations, and the activity of the gene gave the cell its cancerous properties. Temin's hypothesis gave rise to the notion of an oncogene, a gene that could determine whether a cell is normal or cancerous. As this idea developed in many laboratories, it was further suggested that an oncogene might be present in an inactive form in normal cells and activated in some way in cancer cells, or alternatively an oncogene could be brought into the cell by a virus. The actual discovery of oncogenes was a result of combining new technologies of molecular genetics, molecular biology, and cell biology to seek these predicted genes. This discovery was perhaps the most important occurrence in cancer research in recent years, for it is providing the beginnings of an understanding of growth regulation in normal cells and the first hints of the nature of transformation of a normal cell. The mid-1980s is an exciting time for cancer biology, because new information is becoming available at an extraordinary rate, and for the first time one can see a path to understanding malignancy in terms of gene function. Unfortunately, at this time we have no definitive answers to present in this chapter, which instead is more a collection of observations. In a few years many answers will surely be available, and a rewriting of this book will be essential.

RETROVIRUSES

In 1911 Peyton Rous of the Rockefeller Institute in New York found that chicken cells could be transformed into cancer cells by an extract from chicken tumors that had been filtered to remove all cells and major cellular material. He concluded that a virus, thousands of times smaller than cells and able to pass through the finest filters available, was responsible for the transformation. The scientific community of the early 1900s was not ready to accept the notion of a cancer virus (Rous himself abandoned the study of the virus in 1915), and the discovery was not appreciated until the 1960s when (1) the virus was seen by electron microscopy and (2) virus-induced transformation of normal cells to cancer cells was carried out in the laboratory. The virus has since been named Rous sarcoma virus, commonly abbreviated RSV. Rous was awarded the Nobel Prize in 1966, after the longest time interval between discovery and award in the history of the Nobel Prize.

Rous sarcoma virus contains no DNA and uses RNA as its genetic material. An important discovery made in the 1960s was that chick cells transformed to cancer cells by RSV contain DNA sequences complementary to the base sequence of RSV RNA. Furthermore, a variety of experiments showed that these sequences are incorporated into the chromosome of the chick DNA. This observation was a clear violation of the dogma that DNA makes RNA, since no mechanism was known for using RNA as a template for DNA synthesis. Rous sarcoma virus (and several related viruses) was then placed in a separate group called retroviruses (retro: Latin, backwards). The search for the RNA-to-DNA mechanism led to the discovery of the enzyme reverse transcriptase in the laboratories of David Baltimore and Howard Temin, both of whom were awarded the Nobel Prize in 1975 for this work. Reverse transcriptase is contained in the virus particle. When RSV infects a cell, both viral RNA and reverse transcriptase enter the cell. The enzyme copies the viral RNA, producing DNA, and later the DNA is inserted into the DNA of the host cell (Figure 8-1). There the DNA serves as a template for synthesis of the messenger RNA molecules needed to produce progeny virus, which are released from the cell at a later time, without destruction of the cell. This RNA-to-DNA conversion and the insertion of the DNA are an integral part of the reproductive cycle of the virus. How the virus (and related viruses) reproduce is of little concern to cancer biology. What is important are the following features of most retroviruses: (1) Virus-derived DNA becomes part of the chromosome of the cell and hence is carried through from generation to generation as the cell multiplies; that is, a cell transformed by a retrovirus to a tumor cell produces progeny cells that are all tumor cells. (2) Viral genes become part of the collection of genes active in the cell, and some of these genes can convert an immortalized, but noncancerous, cell to a cancer cell; such a gene is called an oncogene. The oncogene present in Rous sarcoma virus will be described shortly.

Since the discovery of Rous sarcoma virus hundreds of RNA tumor viruses have been isolated from tumors in many species of animals. These viruses induce a variety of sarcomas, leukemias, and carcinomas. Each virus is able to convert viral RNA to DNA and to insert the newly made DNA into the host chromosome. Furthermore, transformation of infected cells to cancer cells requires both integration and the function of a particular gene. As will be seen in a later section, there are numerous viral oncogenes, but each viral species does not carry a unique oncogene; that is, many oncogenes are present in several different viruses. We will see also that in many cases the viral oncogene resembles a normal cellular gene.

DNA TUMOR VIRUSES

A number of viruses containing DNA also cause tumors. The three that have been studied most extensively are polyoma virus (the first

DNA tumor virus discovered), SV40, and adenovirus. These viruses also insert DNA into the chromosome of cells and thereby cause transformation. No RNA intermediate is required for insertion. Polyoma and SV40 insert the entire viral DNA molecule, but adenoviruses usually insert only a fragment. In each case, transformation requires the activity of particular genes. The activity of the genes of polyoma

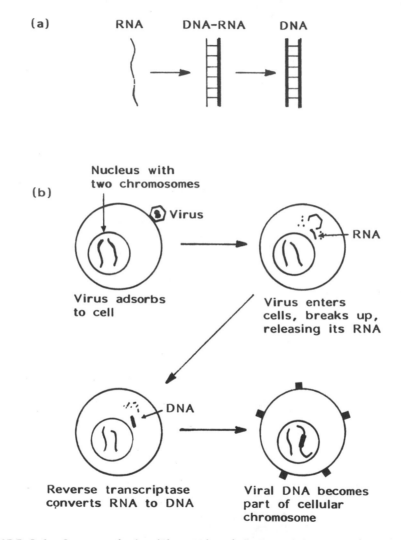

FIGURE 8-1 Stages of the life cycle of Rous sarcoma virus important to cancer biology. (a) RNA is copied by reverse transcriptase, yielding DNA. (b) Conversion of viral RNA to viral DNA, and integration of viral DNA into the cellular chromosome. Tumor-specific antigens (■) appear on the cell surface after integration.

and SV40 is made evident by the physical presence of the proteins synthesized by the genes in the nucleus of the cell. The products are called T antigens (T for tumor, and antigen because they are usually detected by immunological tests). The molecular biology of the T antigens is complex, because there are several gene products and because the proteins have several enzymatic and regulatory activities. Thus, these proteins will not be described in any detail. Suffice it to say that the T antigens bind to DNA and initiate DNA replication, which is probably their major function in the life cycle of the viruses; however, whether this property is required for transformation is controversial. What is clear is that viral transformation by the DNA tumor viruses involves a complex interplay between host genes and viral genes, which is at present quite poorly understood. We will see that the function of the oncogenes of the RNA tumor viruses, though still obscure, may be a little less complex.

THE ONCOGENE OF ROUS SARCOMA VIRUS

The oncogene of Rous sarcoma virus was first detected by the discovery of an interesting mutation in the virus. In Chapter 2 it was pointed out that a single base substitution in DNA may result in the production of a mutant protein with an amino acid sequence that differs from that of the normal protein; the altered amino acid sequence causes aberrant folding of the protein molecule, leading to a reduction or loss of biological activity. There are many types of mutations, and one that has been quite useful is the temperature-sensitive mutation. Such a mutation yields a protein with an altered amino acid sequence, but the folding, and hence the biological activity, is normal at standard temperatures and abnormal only at elevated temperatures. That is, a cell with a temperature-sensitive mutation may behave completely normally at one temperature, yet die, or least be defective, at another. Mutations of this type have been isolated in many viruses; they are detected by the ability of the virus to multiply below a critical temperature (at permissive temperatures) and the failure to multiply above that temperature (at nonpermissive temperatures).

In 1970 a temperature-sensitive mutation was isolated in Rous sarcoma virus, which only affects the ability to transform chicken cells. The mutant virus reproduces over a wide range of temperatures, yet above a certain temperature (about 35°C) cells are not transformed. At both permissive and nonpermissive temperatures the viral RNA is still converted to viral DNA by reverse transcriptase, and the DNA is integrated. These results show that even though integration is essential for transformation, it is not sufficient. An important experiment with this mutant was the following. Cells were infected at a low (permissive) temperature, transformation was allowed to take place by permitting continued cell division at the low temperature, and then the temperature was raised to a nonpermissive temperature. The transformed cells reacquired the growth characteristics of normal cells (Figure 8-2). The interpretation of the experiment was the following. The gene in which the mutation had occurred makes a protein that is essential for transformation. When the protein produced by the mutant gene is active (low temperature), cells containing the protein are transformed; but when the protein is inactive (high temperature), cells were normal, even if they have previously been transformed. Thus, it was concluded that continued activity of the gene is necessary to maintain the transformed state.

This temperature–sensitive mutation was located in a gene that had not previously been recognized. It was named src (for sarcoma). It plays no role in reproduction of the virus but is responsible for converting normal cells to cancer cells. By use of genetic engineering techniques a variant of Rous sarcoma virus was created that completely lacked the src gene. This "deletion" mutant again retained the ability to multiply (showing unambiguously that the gene is nonessential) but could not transform normal cells. In an exciting experiment a fragment of viral DNA containing only the src gene was also isolated and added to cultured chick cells; when this fragment alone was incorporated into the chromosome of a normal cell, the cell was transformed. Thus, the src gene is a cancer gene (an oncogene). In a later section we will discuss whether presence of an oncogene, though necessary for

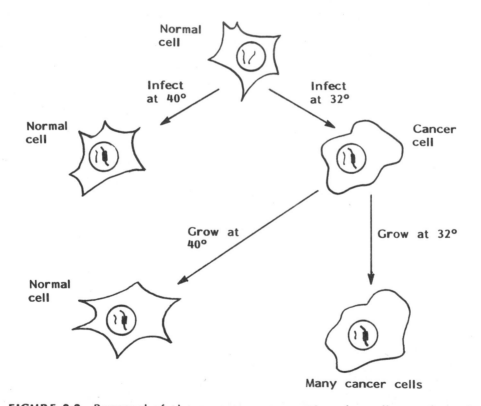

FIGURE 8-2 Reversal of the cancerous properties of a cell transformed by a Rous sarcoma virus mutant with a temperature-sensitive mutation in the src gene. The heavy bar in the nucleus represents viral DNA integrated into one of the chromosomes.

transformation, is sufficient (recall the two-step theory of cancer discussed in Chapters 5 and 7).

The product of the src gene is a single protein called pp60-v-src; the 60 refers to the fact that its molecular weight is 60,000 (which is not important), and v indicates that the gene is derived from a virus (a distinction that will soon be seen to be important). The protein is an enzyme that is able to add a phosphate group to the amino acid tyrosine in cellular proteins. An enzyme that adds phosphates to a protein is called a protein kinase. Most enzymes of this sort act on the amino acid serine; the src enzyme is unusual in its preference for tyrosine and is called a tyrosine-specific protein kinase. Similar enzymes have been found to be the products of the transforming genes of other retroviruses.

Protein kinases are common enzymes in animal cells. They function mainly as regulators of the activity of other proteins by adding a phosphate group (phosphorylation) to an amino acid. For some proteins, addition of the phosphate brings out enzymatic activity of the protein, whereas for other proteins phosphorylation has an inactivating effect. A given protein kinase is usually able to phosphorylate a large number of proteins, so the regulatory activity of these kinases can be quite far-reaching. It is easy to imagine that the synthesis of an enzyme like the src protein kinase could change the growth properties of a cell in a dramatic way, for it could activate or inactivate a large number of enzymes, some of which could be involved in growth regulation. Studies with temperature-sensitive mutants of oncogenes in many retroviruses have shown that tyrosine kinase activity and transformation go hand in hand. At permissive temperatures the tyrosine kinase activity is evident, cells are transformed, and some cellular proteins contain phosphorylated tyrosine. At nonpermissive temperatures there is neither tyrosine kinase activity nor transformation, and there are no phosphorylated tyrosines.

It is obvious that to understand the significance of the kinase activity, the essential proteins that are phosphorylated must be identified. Many proteins that are phosphorylated by the src kinase have been isolated, but the functions of most of these proteins have not yet been identified. Some information about these proteins will be given in a later section.

ONCOGENES IN CANCER CELLS

Recognition that a single gene such as src could cause transformation led to a search for oncogenes in cancer cells obtained by surgical excision from cancer patients. Recall that the src gene can cause transformation in two ways: by integration into a chromosome of an entire Rous sarcoma virus DNA molecule or a fragment of DNA containing only the src gene. The latter result suggested that it might be possible to find an oncogene in a cancer cell by testing DNA fragments isolated from human cancers for their ability to transform a cultured normal cell. Such experiments were carried out independently in several laboratories, using slightly different systems. These experiments will surely be considered some day (if not already) to be one of the greatest steps forward in cancer research.

The first experiment, which used newly developed techniques of genetic engineering, utilized DNA from a line of human bladder cancer cells (Figure 8-3). The DNA was fragmented and added to a culture of mouse cells (strain 3T3, a cell line used repeatedly in such studies). The result of this simple experiment was that some of the mouse cells were transformed, which indicated that an oncogene was present in the bladder cancer cells. In a second experiment the DNA fragments were separated into a large number of fractions and each was tested for transforming activity. It was found that only a single DNA fragment could induce the transformation. Therefore, this fragment contained the human bladder cancer oncogene. (Another set of experiments used human lymphoma cells, and a lymphoma oncogene was isolated.)

Once the human bladder oncogene was discovered, the question of where it came from was raised immediately. According to the mutational theory of cancer discussed in Chapter 3, the bladder oncogene should be a mutant form of a normal gene. Indeed this is the case, for it was possible to isolate from normal bladder cells a DNA fragment whose coding sequence contains a base sequence that differs from the bladder oncogene in only one base: a guanine in the normal DNA is replaced by a thymine in the oncogene. Thus, for this particular human bladder cancer, the oncogene is a mutant form of a normal gene. Similar results have been obtained for several, but not all oncogenes.

THE CELLULAR COUNTERPART OF THE src GENE

The discovery that the bladder oncogene has a counterpart in normal cells suggested that the src gene of Rous sarcoma virus might also have a counterpart in normal cells. Another point raised this possibility. A search for a src-like gene was made in the DNA of chickens and other birds, again using techniques of genetic engineering. A similar base sequence was found; what is more, it was then also found in the DNA of fishes, mammals, and humans! In fact, it appears that all vertebrates possess DNA sequences similar to that of the src gene. To distinguish the two classes of sequences, the viral sequence has been renamed v-src, and the cellular sequence is called c-src. The protein made by c-src is also a tyrosine kinase, but its enzymatic activity is less than 10 percent that of the v-src kinase.

Two simple possibilities have been suggested for the origin of c-src and v-src: (1) c-src arose in a wide variety of organisms by repeated infection of these organisms with retroviruses through evolutionary time, that is, c-src is a derivative of v-src; (2) v-src was somehow picked up by the virus from cellular DNA in an event that provided the virus with the tumor-forming ability (v-src is a derivative of c-src). The fact that Rous sarcoma virus can multiply without the src gene (that is, that the gene is unnecessary to the virus) suggests that the second explanation may be correct, and study of the structure of c-src and v-src provided verification. Viral genes usually consist of uninterrupted coding sequences, whereas genes in animal cells often contain noncoding interruptions, called <u>intervening</u> <u>sequences</u> or <u>introns</u> (Figure 8-4). Analysis of the base sequences of these genes has shown that <u>c-src</u> sequences are always interrupted and <u>v-src</u> sequences are never interrupted. Since there are many examples of loss of introns and none of acquisition of introns, it has been concluded that <u>v-src</u> was acquired from a cell containing <u>c-src</u>

Human bladder cancer isolated

↓

DNA isolated from cancer

↓

Bladder cancer DNA fragmented

↓

Fragments added to culture of mouse 3T3 cells

↓

Some of the mouse cells take up the DNA fragments,
    and some of the DNA becomes integrated into a
    mouse chromosome

↓

Some mouse cells are transformed

FIGURE 8-3 Flow chart for the first experiment that demonstrated an oncogene in cells of a naturally occurring cancer.

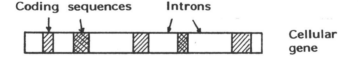

Coding sequences   Introns

Cellular
gene

Viral
gene

FIGURE 8-4 Differences between cellular protooncogenes and viral oncogenes. The cellular gene contains noncoding introns (these are excised from messenger RNA before protein synthesis occurs). The viral gene has the same coding sequence as the cellular gene but without interruptions. Different segments of the coding sequence are shown with different types of cross-hatching only for the purpose of identifying corresponding regions.

at some time in the past, and that in the virus the introns served no purpose, so were eventually deleted by repeated mutation. The presence of c-src in a wide variety of vertebrates suggests that c-src is an essential gene of these animals, probably having a regulatory role in the development of normal organisms.

Other retrovirus genes have counterparts in cellular DNA. In each case, the cellular genes are interrupted by intervening sequences and hence have the structure of typical cellular genes. It seems to be a general phenomenon that retroviruses picked up their oncogenes from normal (and probably essential) cellular genes. Such cellular genes are called protooncogenes.

The bladder oncogene differs from its protooncogene by a single base. It is of theoretical importance to know whether this is a general phenomenon or if the sequence of the cellular counterpart could be identical to that of the oncogene. In fact, both types of pairs of oncogenes and protooncogenes have been observed. When the sequences do differ, one may conclude that the protooncogene does not by itself cause transformation and a mutation produces the cancerous form. However, when the sequences are identical, one must explain how the gene can be harmless in a normal cell, yet so dangerous in a cancer cell. A variety of hypotheses have been made, only some of which are supported to any extent by experiment results. One possibility is that a single copy of the protooncogene is harmless, but when a cell has an extra copy (provided by the integrated viral DNA), the doubling of the amount of gene product puts cell growth and division out of control. This is not unreasonable, especially since very frequently several copies of the viral DNA are integrated. Another possibility, which we will see is true in some cases, is that the amount of protein made by the viral oncogene is much greater than that made by the cellular gene, either because the viral gene is regulated in a different way or because the viral gene has a different location from the cellular gene. These possibilities will be discussed in a later section of this chapter.

CARCINOGENS AND ONCOGENES

At one time it was believed that all cancers arose from viral genes that are contained in normal cells and that are activated by chemical carcinogens and radiation. The evidence supporting this view was that many agents that induce transformation also cause retrovirus particles to appear in animal cell cultures. The conclusion was that many cells harbor latent retroviruses and, in a way that is not clear, these viruses are activated by carcinogens. Whereas it is possible that some cancers are caused in this way, after many years of trying to prove this hypothesis, strong support has never been obtained. Furthermore, a great many cancers, especially human cancers, show no evidence either for virus production or participation of viruses in any way, and in a large number of experiments in which normal cells are treated with carcinogens and transformation occurs, virus particles are not seen.

Many carcinogens are mutagens (Chapter 6), which suggests that a carcinogen might act by causing a mutation in a protooncogene, thereby converting it to an oncogene. As a test of this hypothesis, the following experiment has recently been done. Rats were treated with the carcinogen nitrosomethylurea, and mammary carcinomas formed in many of the rats. Tumors were excised, and the DNA was isolated from the cancer cells and fragmented. This DNA was then added to cultures of mouse 3T3 cells (as in the original experiment that demonstrated the existence of the bladder oncogene) to test for transformation. Indeed, transformed cells resulted. Analysis of the DNA used showed that the transforming DNA contained a rat mammary oncogene. A counterpart was sought and found in normal rat tissue. Determination of the base sequences of the mammary oncogene and the cellular gene gave two remarkable results: (1) the mammary protooncogene and the bladder protooncogene had the same sequence, and (2) the mammary oncogene differed from its normal counterpart by a single base, which was at the same position as the altered base in the bladder cancer oncogene. Thus, it could be concluded that (1) the cancers in the human bladder and in the rat mammary gland were caused by mutations of the same gene, and (2) the carcinogen that caused the mammary cancer in the rat had mutated the normal gene. Since this experiment was done, numerous examples of mutation of a gene by a carcinogen to form an oncogene have been observed. At this time there are about 20 different oncogenes known, which appear repeatedly, as will be seen in the following section. In a later section, we will see that many oncogenes have the same coding sequences as their cellular counterparts.

RELATION BETWEEN ANIMAL AND VIRAL ONCOGENES

If oncogenes are altered forms (or aberrantly expressed forms) of normal genes that usually participate in growth regulation, it seems likely that the number of different oncogenes should be fairly small. Thus, we should expect that if a large number of tumor viruses and tumors are screened for oncogenes, the same ones should appear repeatedly. In the preceding section, one example of this was seen: the oncogene in human bladder carcinoma is the same as that in rat mammary carcinoma. Furthermore, recall that the two oncogenes were obtained from human and rat tumors but tested in mouse 3T3 cells; since these oncogenes transformed the mouse cells, the ability of an oncogene to transform cells crosses species barriers (at least in mammals), suggesting that growth regulation in all mammals may have common features. Note also the possibility, raised by the presence of c-src in normal tissue, that viruses and normal cells may carry the same set of oncogenes and protooncogenes.

   To see whether the number of oncogenes is indeed small, oncogenes were isolated from a large number of viruses and cancerous human tissue, and their counterparts were isolated from normal tissue. The base sequences of all of these genes were determined. The first evidence for commonality came from a study of the oncogene originally detected in Kirsten sarcoma virus, which causes sarcoma in rats. This oncogene, named ras (rat sarcoma), was also found in Harvey sarcoma virus. Except for a single base change, the ras sequence was the same as that reported above for human bladder carcinoma and was also found in human lung and colon carcinomas! A similar sequence but with a different base change was found in a human neuroblastoma and a fibrosarcoma. This variant was called N-ras. Studies of a large number of viruses and tumors (human cancers of colon, lung, pancreas, skin, breast, brain, and white cells, and a variety of rat and mouse tumors) has led to the identification of more than 20 different oncogenes, which are listed in Table 8-1. Their curious names are all abbreviations or acronyms for the virus or tissue of origin. Analysis of the activities of their gene products shows that several are tyrosine kinases (like src), two are threonine kinases (putting a phosphate group on the amino acid threonine), a few are simply proteins that bind tightly to DNA, a some have features in common with growth factors (discussed later in the chapter).

ONCOGENES AND TWO-STEP INDUCTION OF CANCER

In the experiments and tests described so far, the presence of an active oncogene seems to be able to confer cancerous properties on a cell. This fact is in conflict with the arguments given in earlier chapters that induction of cancer requires at least two steps, initiation and promotion. The key to understanding this apparent paradox is noting that all tests for oncogenic potential have been made with an established line of cells obtained from a mouse, namely, 3T3 cells. This cell line, which had been maintained for thousands of generations, was chosen because it had been used for many years to study viral transformation and chemical carcinogenesis. The 3T3 line became popular for these studies because it was easily transformed. A little thought should suggest to the reader that 3T3 cells probably already experienced the initiation step, a logical conclusion since 3T3 cells grow indefinitely in culture and hence have been immortalized.

With this in mind, the two-step hypothesis could be tested in culture by determining whether a known oncogene could transform other cells that had not been immortalized. Studies with freshly isolated normal skin cells (not yet immortalized) of a mouse indicated that these cells could not be transformed in culture with purified ras DNA. In a second experiment portions of the skin cell culture were treated either with x rays or a chemical carcinogen, and a few immortalized cell lines were isolated from these treated cells. These newly immortalized cells were then tested with ras DNA, and it was found that ras could transform these cells. Thus, ras, or more precisely, the ras gene product, is a promoter. Studies with several different oncogenes gave similar results.

Some retroviral oncogenes are responsible for cancer in animals yet do not test as oncogenes with mouse 3T3 cells. A possible explanation is that these oncogenes are initiators rather than promoters, which seems to apply to an oncogene called myc, found in a chicken leukemia virus. Myc does not transform 3T3 cells, yet induces transformation of normal cells at a low frequency. However, normal skin cells can be transformed by sequential treatment first with myc DNA and then with ras DNA. In other words, myc substitutes for the x rays or the chemical carcinogen and acts as an initiator; ras is the promoter. Indeed, myc functions to immortalize cells, as expected of an initiator. We mentioned earlier that the cancer-causing potential of the DNA tumor viruses, polyoma virus and adenovirus, is more complex than that of the retroviruses. Recognition that there are two types of oncogenes, initiator and promoter oncogenes, has made transformation by these viruses more understandable. These viruses carry several oncogenes, for example, large T, small t, and middle t for polyoma. Large T antigen and an adenovirus oncogene called EIA, like myc, have an initiator function; the polyoma middle t antigen and the adenovirus EIB oncogene, like ras, have a promoter function. The DNA virus genes that function like myc do not all have the same base sequence as myc, which indicates that different genes can immortalize cells. Similarly, the genes with the promoter function do not all have the base sequence of ras. Since a variety of oncogenes transform 3T3 (that is, have promoter function), it is clear that many different events in a cell can cause the final step in conversion of an immortalized cell to a cancer cell.

TABLE 8-1 Some oncogenes and their sources

Oncogene	Source*
abl	Mouse leukemia, human leukemia cells
B-lym	Chicken and human lymphoma cells
erbA	Chicken leukemia
erbB	Chicken leukemia
ets	Chicken leukemia
fes	Cat sarcoma
fgr	Cat sarcoma
fms	Cat sarcoma
fos	Mouse sarcoma
fps	Chicken sarcoma
Ha-ras	Rat sarcoma; human and rat carcinoma cells
Ki-ras	Rat sarcoma; human carcinoma, sarcoma, and leukemia cells
mil	Chicken sarcoma
mos	Mouse sarcoma, mouse leukemia cell
myb	Chicken leukemia and human leukemia cells
myc	Chicken leukemia; human lymphoma cells
N-ras	Human leukemia and carcinoma cells
raf	Mouse sarcoma
rel	Turkey leukemia
ros	Chicken sarcoma
sis	Monkey sarcoma
ski	Chicken sarcoma
src	Chicken sarcoma
yes	Chicken sarcoma

*Indicates a retrovirus unless indicated as a cell.

ACTIVATION OF ONCOGENES

We have pointed out that counterparts to oncogenes are found in normal cells and that often the distinction between a normal gene and an oncogene is a single base pair, in which case the oncogene is a mutant form of the normal gene. Although we have no information about the biological function of the oncogene products, it is worth considering the kinds of events that might take place:

1. A single base change could cause activation by increasing or decreasing the activity of the oncogene protein. For example, if the protein were a regulatory gene whose job is to turn on synthesis of a growth protein, increased activity of the oncogene product could result in excess synthesis of the growth protein. On the other hand, the oncogene product could have the job of turning <u>off</u> synthesis of a growth inhibitor; in this case, inactivation of the oncogene protein would eliminate its inhibitory activity, and excess growth protein would be made.
2. Another possibility is that the oncogene protein is a growth-stimulating molecule, whose activity is regulated by other (unknown) proteins. A change in the oncogene protein (caused by the base pair change) could cause a loss of its ability to respond to the regulator; in this case, the growth-stimulating activity of the oncogene product could become excessive.
3. The oncogene protein might be unstable, with its activity regulated by the relative rates of synthesis and degradation of the protein. An alteration in its structure might prevent or reduce its rate of degradation, without affecting its biochemical activity. In this case, its total activity in the cell would increase.

When an oncogene does not differ from its cellular counterpart, the hypothetical mechanisms for oncogene action listed above do not necessarily apply. In studies of cell biology it has become abundantly clear that certain biological functions are determined not simply by the presence of a particular gene product, but by the concentration of the product. This raises the possibility that the conversion of a protooncogene to an active oncogene, thereby inducing the cancerous state, is occurring simply by changes in concentration. We now consider how a change in concentration might come about and also provide some evidence that this does occur in some cases.

The amount of a gene product contained in a cell is determined by its rate of synthesis (also, its rate of degradation, but this possibility will not be considered here). The rate of synthesis of most proteins is determined by the rate of synthesis of the messenger RNA encoding the protein. A variety of features of DNA structure affect the synthesis of messenger RNA. For simplicity, we shall consider only two: promoter strength and regulatory regions. The region of a DNA molecule at which RNA polymerase, the enzyme responsible for synthesizing RNA, binds and initiates RNA synthesis is called a <u>promoter</u>. This region is little more than a sequence of a few tens of bases that provides both a binding site and signals to start polymerization. There are many, possibly hundreds, of different promoter sequences, each yielding different rates of RNA synthesis. Adjacent to the promoter, there are often (but not always) regulatory sequences that determine (1) whether RNA polymerase is able to bind to the promoter or (2) how efficiently binding occurs. Without going into any detail, we can say that the number of copies of a particular protein is primarily determined by base sequences adjacent to the gene encoding that protein. Therefore, and this is the essential point, the activity of a gene can be changed by altering the adjacent promoter and/or regulatory sequences. Indeed, this phenomenon has been observed. That is, some oncogenes differ from the normal counterparts only in that base changes exist in the promoter, and these changes presumably alter the rate of messenger RNA synthesis.

Another important mechanism by which the expression of a protooncogene can be altered is by moving the gene to a new location, for example, by relocating it next to a different promoter, or by separating it from an adjacent regulatory element. This is presumably one way by which a protooncogene becomes oncogenic when located in a virus. That is, a promoter in the virus may have a significantly different strength from the promoter adjacent to a protooncogene in a normal cell. Thus, when the viral DNA is inserted into the chromosome of an infected cell, the viral oncogene may be expressed at a much greater rate than the protooncogene, which is still at its normal location (Figure 8-5). A particular feature of virus structure is important in this regard. Many viruses contain special sequences called enhancers. These are activating sequences that cause a very high rate of RNA synthesis. By genetic engineering it has been possible to isolate these enhancer sequences and place a variety of genes next to them. In most cases the synthesis of messenger RNA increases about 100-fold. These enhancers could cause synthesis of huge amounts of oncogene messenger RNA and hence of oncogene proteins.

A variety of experiments have been carried out that indicate that relocating a protooncogene can convert it to an oncogene. For example, using techniques of genetic engineering the normal mouse protooncogene, c-ras (and another called c-mos), has been attached to a viral regulatory sequence, without any alteration of the base sequence of the oncogene itself, as is the case with v-ras. This constructed DNA thereby gained the ability to transform mouse 3T3 cells. In another experiment a DNA fragment containing a protooncogene was isolated, and the terminal sequences, which presumably contained the regulatory elements that are adjacent to the gene, were removed; the protooncogene also gained the ability to transform 3T3 cells.

Recall from Chapters 4 and 7 that chromosome changes are common in cancers. The most common type of change is translocation, a chromosome alteration in which two chromosomes have apparently exchanged segments. For example, in Burkitt's lymphoma, fragments in chromosomes 8 and 14 are exchanged in 90% of the patients, between chromosomes 8 and 2 in 5% of the patients, and between chromosomes 8 and 22 in another 5%. Note that in each case a segment of chromosome

8 has been moved. The protooncogene c-myc corresponding to the oncogene of Burkitt's lymphoma, v-myc, is located on chromosome 8. In each of the translocations, c-myc is relocated adjacent to a gene encoding an antibody. This relocation apparently places the protooncogene under control of the genes that regulate antibody synthesis, so that c-myc is made in large quantities. Numerous examples of translocations of protooncogenes have been observed. Recall that patients with chronic myelogenous leukemia have a translocation between chromosomes 22 and 9. This causes the protooncogene abl (also present as the oncogene of Abelson mouse leukemia virus) to move from its normal location in chromosome 9 to chromosome 22; at this new location the rate of synthesis of c-abl messenger RNA is 8-fold greater than when the gene is in chromosome 9.

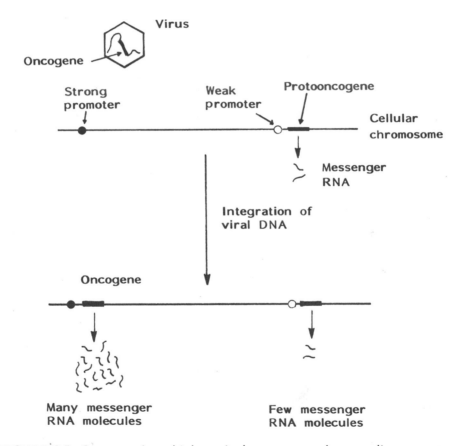

FIGURE 8-5 One way by which a viral oncogene whose coding sequence is the same as that of its cellular counterpart could produce excess product. The viral gene is adjacent to a stronger promoter than the cellular gene; an alternative is that the strong promoter could be present in the viral DNA itself.

One must not be misled in thinking that simply increasing the amount of messenger RNA of a particular protooncogene is sufficient to induce cancer (recall that two steps are required to induce cancer). In fact, in several experiments synthesis of messenger RNA of a protooncogene has been amplified by genetic engineering and malignant transformation does not occur, clearly indicating a requirement for other events, which remain to be discovered.

ONCOGENE PROTEINS

Oncogenes and protooncogenes encode proteins, and certainly the activity of these proteins must be involved in transformation. In this section we examine several classes of oncogene proteins (Table 8-2), including, when possible, how they might work.

Protein Kinases

Earlier in this chapter we indicated that several oncogenes encode protein kinases, specifically those that place phosphate groups on tyrosine or threonine. The main approach to understanding how the kinase activity leads to transformation has been to seek proteins that contain phosphorylated tyrosines or threonines and see what these proteins do. These studies have not led to any detailed understanding of the transformation process but do indicate why some of the changes that accompany transformation come about. One of the first such proteins identified is p36, a protein found in cells infected with Rous sarcoma virus. It is located on the inner (cytoplasmic) side of the cell membrane. In some cell types it is involved in some way with anchoring of microfilaments. Recall that cancer cells have disorganized microfilaments. Another protein whose tyrosines are phosphorylated is vinculin, a protein present in small patches (adhesion plaques) on the cell surface. These patches help cells adhere to surfaces and to one another and serve as attachment sites for bundles of microfilaments. Phosphorylated vinculin is less able to organize the microfilaments. Possibly, this alteration of vinculin is responsible for

TABLE 8-2 Class of oncogene proteins

Protein	Oncogene
Tyrosine kinase	abl, fes, fgr, fps, ros, src, yes
Other protein kinases	erbB, fms, mil, mos, raf
Nuclear proteins	B-lym, fos, myb, myc, ski
Growth factor	sis
GTP-binding proteins	Ha-ras, Ki-ras, N-ras

the decreased adhesion (a malignant feature) of cancer cells and the fact that cancer cells are usually rounder than normal cells. The src kinase has also been observed to phosphorylate a lipid (a nonprotein molecule related to fats) called phosphatidylinositol, which is contained in the cell membrane. The altered lipid is then cleaved into two substances, diacylglycerol and triphosphoinositide (the names need not be remembered). Diacylglycerol activates another protein kinase that puts phosphate groups on the amino acid serine, and thereby causes alteration of a very large number of proteins. The other fragment, causes a release of calcium bound in the membranes. The significance of this release is not clear, but recall from Chapter 4 that one of the growth features of cancer cells involves calcium. Both of these events could alter the control of cell division and other events occurring in transformation.

Growth Factors

In Chapter 4 we discussed a variety of substances that affect the growth rate of particular cell types; some of these are called growth factors. Recently a connection has been seen between certain oncogenes and growth factors. The v-erbB oncogene is carried by a chicken retrovirus that causes red blood cell leukemia (avian erythroblastosis virus). It is a large gene, part of which encodes a tyrosine protein kinase. However, of possibly greater interest is the other part of the protein, which is closely related to the cell surface receptor for epidermal growth factor (EGF). The normal receptor, which is believed to be encoded in the cellular counterpart, c-erbB, is a large protein that spans the cell membrane. Only a portion of the receptor (the part inside the membrane and inside the cell) is encoded by v-erbB. It is thought that when v-erbB was acquired by the virus, only a part of the c-erbB gene was picked up. It is possible that the altered receptor produced by v-erbB disrupts the regulatory mechanisms in which the receptor is a crucial link. Interestingly, when EGF binds to the altered receptor, the tyrosine kinase is activated. The reader surely must have the impression that we are seeing in these observations something very significant, yet still well hidden.

The oncogene sis, which is carried by simian sarcoma virus, encodes a protein similar to the platelet-derived growth factor (PDGF), which is made by the protooncogene c-sis. Cells infected with simian sarcoma virus continually produce the altered PDGF, which binds to the receptors on the cell surface. Not all cells produce the PDGF receptor. Possibly, transformation only occurs when a cell that already makes the receptor is infected with the virus. This could cause autostimulation of cell division. Experimental confirmation of these hypotheses is not yet available.

The ras Proteins

An underlying theme in biology is that fundamental processes are usually carried out in much the same way for all organisms, though there are subtle differences between the prokaryotes (cells without true nuclei, such as bacteria), and the eukaryotes (cells with true nuclei). For example, all organisms use DNA and RNA polymerases to make DNA and RNA, glycolysis is a a universal reaction for metabolizing glucose, and the mechanisms for protein synthesis differ only in detail between prokaryotes and eukaryotes. Since cell division is a property of all cells, one would expect some common features in the mechanism and regulation of this division.

Studies of cell division in bacteria have progressed at a more rapid rate than with animal cells, since in a given time period bacteria divide about 50 times more often than animal cells in culture. Also, bacteria have only a single chromosome, so the mechanism is probably simpler than the complex mitotic system of animal cells. An inherent difference between multiplication of bacteria and animal cells is that bacteria multiply continually, whereas animal cells organized in tissue do not. The yeasts (and other single cell eukaryotes), however, are in an intermediate situation: they are free-living organisms like bacteria, but they are nonetheless eukaryotes with many chromosomes. Since the prokaryotes and the eukaryotes diverged hundreds of millions of years ago, one may hope that certain systems that regulate cell division in animal cells may have counterparts in yeast. If so, one would have an experimental handle on the regulation of cell division, because yeast cells can be manipulated experimentally with much greater ease than animal cells. Recently, analogues of src and ras have been detected in fruit flies and in ordinary baker's yeast. Yeast has two ras genes. Inactivation of both genes by mutation prevents growth; either gene in active form is sufficient for normal growth. One of the most exciting findings of the mid 1980s was the discovery that growth of a yeast that contains two defective ras genes, is restored by uptake of human DNA containing the human c-ras gene. This gives credence to the hypothesis that c-ras is a gene that regulates growth and division in animal cells. Interestingly, only the protooncogene will correct the defect in yeast; none of the altered forms, such as those with a different single base change present in various retroviruses, can substitute for a defective yeast gene. These observations are so recent that little is yet known about the functioning of the normal yeast ras genes. However, a tantalizing observation is that the normal ras protein activates adenylate synthetase, the enzyme responsible for synthesis of the general regulator, cyclic AMP (Chapter 4).

ONCOGENES AND CANCER

The study of oncogenes is one of the most rapidly moving fields in molecular and cell biology, and the amount of information is so great that it is difficult to select the material for presentation in a short chapter. One may ask what concluding statements can be made in the present state of infancy of this field. The most solid conclusions, which are unlikely to be altered as more information is gained, are the following: (1) several, possibly only two, steps are needed for transformation; (2) each of the two recognized steps can, at least for some tumors, be carried out by various oncogenes; (3) oncogenes are formed from protooncogenes by mutation or relocation; (4) relocation can occur either by chromosomal exchanges (translocation) or by means of a virus carrier; and (5) oncogene proteins have a variety of biochemical activities. We do not yet know what really makes a cancer cell cancerous nor do we have any idea how to turn off an oncogene or to reverse the effect of oncogene activity; hence, in that sense, even with the enormous amount of information now available, the "cure" for cancer remains elusive. However, optimism may be derived from the belief, supported by evidence from diseases of the past, that rational treatment will follow from understanding. Most workers in the oncogene field are confident that this understanding will come, at least in part, from the study of oncogenes.

ADDITIONAL READINGS

Aaronson, S.A., C.Y. Dunn, N.W. Ellmore, and A. Eva. 1983. "Retroviral onc genes in human neoplasia." Prog. Clin. Biol. Med., 119, 207.

Androphy, E.J. and D.R. Lowy. 1984. J. Amer. Acad. Dermatol., 10, 125.

Astrin, S.H. and P.G. Rothberg. 1983. "Oncogenes and cancer." Cancer Invest., 1, 355.

Bishop, J.M. 1983. "Cancer genes come of age." Cell, 32, 1018.

Bishop, J.M. 1983. "Cellular oncogenes and retroviruses." Ann. Rev. Biochem., 52, 301.

Bishop, J.M. 1982. "Oncogenes." Scient. Amer., March, 80.

Cline, M.H., D.J. Slamon, and J.S. Lipsick. 1984. "Oncogenes: Implications for the diagnosis and treatment of cancer." Ann. Intern. Med., 101, 223.

Cooper, G.M., and M.A. Lane. 1984. "Cellular transforming genes and oncogenesis." Biochim. Biophys. Acta, 738, 9.

Franchini, G. and F. Wong-Staal. 1984. "Retroviruses and retroviral oncogenes: possible role in human neoplasms and aplasias." Prog. Clin. Biol. Res., 148, 153.

Hall, A. 1984. "Oncogenes. Implications for human cancer: a review." J. Roy. Soc. Med., 77, 410.

Heldin, C.H. and B. Westermark. 1984. "Growth factors: mechanism of action and relation to oncogenes." Cell, 37, 9.

Klein, G. and E. Klein. 1984. "Oncogene activation and tumor progression." Carcinogenesis, 5, 429.

Lebowitz, P. 1983. "Oncogenic genes and their potential role in human malignancy." J. Clin. Oncol., 1, 657.

Littlefield, J.W. 1984. "Genes, chromosomes, and cancer." J. Pediatr., 104, 489.

Marx, J.L. 1984. "What do oncogenes do?" Science, 223, 673, 676.

Newmark, P. 1981. "Tyrosine phosphorylation and oncogenes." Nature, 292, 15.

Paul, J. 1984. "Oncogenes." J. Pathol., 143, 1.

Rowley, J.D. 1983. "Human oncogene locations and chromosome aberrations." Nature, 301, 290.

Sharp, P. 1980. "Molecular biology of oncogenes." Cold Spring. Harb. Symp. Quant. Biol., 44, 1305.

Spandidos, D.A. 1983. "Cellular oncogenes, mutation, and cancer." Anticanc. Res., 3, 121.

Weinberg, R.A. 1983. "A molecular basis of cancer." Scient. Amer., Nov. 126.

Weinberg, R.A. 1983. "Transforming genes of tumor cells." Int. Rev. Cytol. (Suppl.), 15, 191.

Weinberg, R.A. 1983. "Alteration of the genomes of tumor cells." Cancer, 51, 1971.

Weiss, R. 1983. "The myc oncogene in man and birds." Nature, 299, 9.

Immunology
and Cancer

In the early 1900s, a surgeon named William Coley injected cancer patients with mixtures of killed bacteria. These "vaccines" caused symptoms in the patients that were characteristic of acute bacterial infection, including high fever and chills. His records show rather conclusively that this treatment resulted in the complete or partial regression of a substantial number of tumors. This method of cancer treatment was ignored for nearly 60 years, because the reasons for Coley's successes were not understood and early work done with radiation therapy and chemotherapy had instead captured the interests of physicians. We now know that Coley's treatment had stimulated the immune system, enabling an activated army of white blood cells to destroy the cancer cells.

We are just beginning to understand the nature of the immune system and its relationship to cancer. However, knowledge of this topic is accumulating rapidly, and immunological approaches against cancer will probably become more prevalent. Because of differences in the molecules on the surface of normal and cancer cells, our immune system can potentially distinguish these two classes of cells and selectively kill the cancer cells. Current standard methods for treating metastatic cancer, such as chemotherapy, are not as selective and usually result in side effects that are poorly tolerated by many individuals. These side effects occur because the chemicals used in chemotherapy damage normal cells as well as cancer cells. The search for a method that selectively destroys cancer cells, leaving normal cells alone, may be fulfilled in the future if immunotherapy of cancer proves to be as successful as many cancer researchers in the field hope.

CELLS OF THE IMMUNE SYSTEM

The immune system is our major defense against infectious organisms. The system consists of many different types of cells, most of which travel throughout our tissues, seeking out and destroying both foreign cells and foreign substances. A molecule that is recognized as foreign and that activates an immune response is called an antigen. Some of these cells produce antibodies, which are proteins that are designed to combine with an antigen. The antigen-antibody reaction is exceedingly specific; an antigen stimulates production of a particular antibody, and the antibody so produced recognizes and combines only with the antigen that stimulated its synthesis. Normal molecules present in the body are not recognized as foreign (they are not antigenic), so it is said that the immune system can distinguish self from nonself. All cells of the immune system are not antibody producers; some attack and ingest foreign cells.

The immune system is very complex and there is no reason to describe it in detail here. Instead we will discuss what is needed to understand its activity against tumor cells. To start, the reader should recall that cancer cells possess surface antigens that are not found on the surface of normal cells, and that these antigens are the basis of the immune reaction. We will talk more about these antigens later in the chapter.

Macrophages and Monocytes

The body has two basic responses to an antigen: the primary response and the secondary response. The primary response occurs when the body encounters an antigen for the first time. It involves (1) a programming of particular cells to make a specific antibody and (2) growth of a small clone of cells that henceforth is able to make that antibody and no other. Only a fairly small amount of antibody is made in a primary response, though it is usually sufficient to prevent the infection from destroying the body. The secondary response occurs when an antigen is encountered a second (or subsequent) time; in this case the clone of cells enlarges, and huge amounts of specific antibody are made. The secondary response is rapid and accounts for our immunity to diseases that we once had.

Two cell types that participate in the primary response are monocytes, which circulate through the body, and macrophages, which reside primarily in tissue. These cells possess surface receptors for a wide variety of antigens (for example, tumor antigens), bind these antigens, and process them for presentation to the set of cells (lymphocytes) that will ultimately be responsible for inactivating or destroying the antigen. Macrophages have a second function that is important in protection against tumors. That is, following exposure of a macrophage to a surface antigen on a tumor cell a complex series of events occurs that results in activation of the macrophage, enabling it to attack a tumor cell directly and cause it to burst (the bursting of a cell is called lysis). The mechanism of this killing is not known in detail, but two events are essential: the tumor cell must be coated with antibody (made by lymphocytes) that can bind to the surface antigens, and the macrophage must actually come in contact with the antibody-coated tumor cell (Figure 9-1). Some experiments have indicated that the macrophage releases locally toxic molecules, but other experiments indicate that portions of the macrophage actually enter the tumor cell and release lysis enzymes.

T Lymphocytes

Most of the cells that constitute the immune system are derived from cells in bone marrow. A type of cell called a stem cell can differentiate in two different ways to form two major classes of cells. In one pathway cells derived from stem cells migrate to the thymus gland where they are converted to T lymphocytes or T cells; later, the T cells migrate to various lymphoid tissues in the body. In the alternative pathway the precursors move to the spleen and certain tissues of the gastrointestinal tract, where they are converted to B lymphocytes or B cells. (They are called B because the phenomenon was first studied in chickens in which the conversion occurs in an organ called the bursa of Fabricius.) Both T cells and B cells are found in the lymph nodes and in the spleen and circulate through the blood stream.

There are several classes of T cells that are relevant to cancer biology. One class is the helper T cell. These cells can respond to

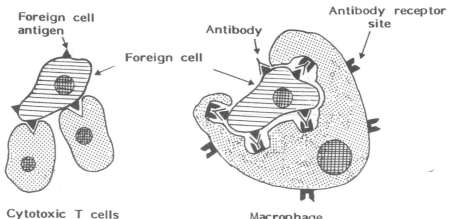

FIGURE 9-1 Modes of destruction of foreign cells, such as tumor cells, by cytotoxic T cells and macrophages. In both cells, surface antigens are recognized. The cytotoxic T cells attack a cell with foreign antigens. The macrophages await binding of antibody to the surface antigens and then engulf any cell that is coated with antibody.

an antigen directly (though macrophages often participate, as explained in the preceding section) by proliferation. In a complex and poorly understood way these cells help other T cells and B cells to function (this will be explained in a moment); they also secrete an activation factor that stimulates macrophages to carry out the cytotoxic function described in the preceding section. A second class of T cells is the effector T cell or cytotoxic killer cell; these cells develop a tumor-killing function when stimulated by a tumor antigen (Figure 9-1). A third category is the suppressor T cell, which modulates the immune response by preventing excessive proliferation of helper T cells and overproduction of antibody by B cells. The balance of activities of the helper T cells and suppressor T cells determines the response of the body to a particular antigen.

B Cells

B cells are responsible for the ultimate synthesis of antibodies. When an animal is exposed to an antigen, the specific helper T cells that proliferate in response to that antigen cause B cells to develop into plasma cells. These cells synthesize the major antibody of the body, immunoglobulin G (IgG), which reacts with the antigen that stimulated the initial response (Figure 9-2). These are the antibodies that destroy bacteria, viruses, and foreign organisms in general. IgG can trigger killing of tumor cells in two ways: complement-induced lysis and antibody-dependent cell-mediated cytoxicity (ADCC). The first mechanism involves a large set of molecules (collectively called complement) that circulate in the blood and in a complicated way cause lysis; it is probably of minor importance in the defense against tumor cells. The ADCC reaction is more significant. This reaction begins with antibody (circulating through the blood and lymph systems or made near the tumor cells) adhering to the tumor antigens on the surface of the tumor cell. Once the IgG is bound to the cell surface, other cells that recognize a specific region of the IgG molecule bind to the tumor cell. These cells, which include macrophages, T cells, and natural killer cells, can cause complete destruction of the tumor cells.

Natural Killer Cells

The natural killer (NK) cells are in the lymphocyte family, but their ability to kill tumor cells does not depend on the synthesis of antibodies to tumor antigens. Precursors to NK cells are stimulated to differentiate into active killer cells by interferons, a class of molecule that is released both by another type of T cell called effector T cells and by active NK cells. Interferon is a primary defense against viral infection, but this role is probably different from that described for tumor cells. Interferon will be discussed in greater detail in Chapter 13.

The reader has surely noted the variety of defenses that the body has against tumor cells and may wonder how tumors ever manage to survive. This will be discussed shortly, after we review the tumor antigens.

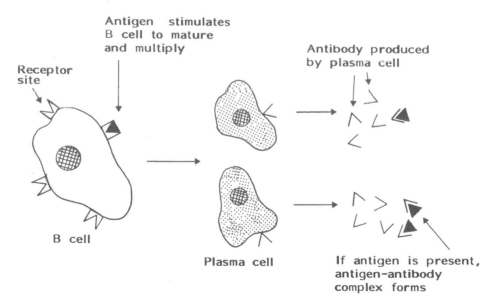

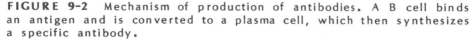

FIGURE 9-2 Mechanism of production of antibodies. A B cell binds an antigen and is converted to a plasma cell, which then synthesizes a specific antibody.

TUMOR ANTIGENS

On numerous occasions we have stated that cancer cells often possess antigens on their cell surfaces that are not present on the surfaces of normal adult cells. These antigens are basically of two types: tumor-associated transplantation antigens (TATA), which appear on the surfaces of cells transformed by viruses or by treatment with chemicals or radiation, and oncodevelopmental antigens (embryonic antigens), which are antigens normally found only on embryonic cells. The antigens induced by viral infection are usually virus-specific rather than tissue-specific, whereas those found on cells transformed by chemical and radiation are usually tissue-specific. The embryonic antigens are often found on spontaneously arising tumors, though they are also present on the surfaces of the cells of many induced tumors. The most commonly observed embryonic antigens are alpha-fetoprotein (AFP), which is found in liver cancers and some cancers of the testis, pancreas, and gastrointestinal tract, and carcinoembryonic antigen (CAE), which is found in cancers of the gastrointestinal tract, pancreas, liver, and lung. AFP is located in fetal cord blood and is produced by fetal liver and the yolk sac. CAE is synthesized by the fetal digestive tract and a variety of epithelial tissues. Neither AFP nor CAE are present at high levels in normal adults, and detection of these proteins in the blood of an adult is usually an indication of a tumor somewhere in the body (liver cancer for AFP, and CAE for intestinal and liver cancer).

A few antigens found in cancer cells are also found in normal adult cells, but in a covered state (Figure 9-3). For example, the S antigen found on the surfaces of cells transformed by SV40 virus is also present in the surfaces of normal cells, but is not exposed. Treatment of normal cells with proteolytic enzymes exposes the S antigen.

NATURAL IMMUNITY TO CANCER AND IMMUNOSURVEILLANCE

Mice can be induced to develop tumors by injection of the carcinogen methylcholanthrene under the skin. Cells from these tumors will grow in other mice of the same strain. If the tumor developing from these inoculated cells is removed from the mouse, that mouse will be resistant to subsequent injections of cells from the same tumor, indicating that the immune system can remember and respond to tumor antigens and destroy tumor cells. Similar observations have been made for tumors induced by viruses. For example, mice became immune to transplants of tumor cells induced by polyoma virus when the mice were inoculated with small amounts of polyoma virus before the tumor cells were injected. Presumably, the virus caused some cell transformation in the mice, but the transformed cells were rejected. In this process, the immune system became alerted to tumor cells transformed by polyoma virus, so when a large dose of these cells was presented, the immune system of the mouse could destroy them.

These findings have given rise to the concept of immune surveillance, an idea that has had many ups and downs in the past 40 years, as new experimental results were obtained. The theory

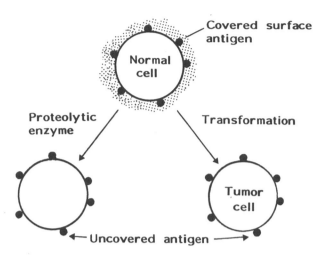

FIGURE 9-3 Demonstration that normal cells often possess tumor antigens on their surfaces but in a covered state. Treatment of certain normal cells with a protein-degrading enzyme exposes some of the same antigens found on transformed cells.

postulates that transformed malignant cells arise frequently in normal individuals and that the cells are usually destroyed by the immune response. An argument given for this theory is the weak immune response found in many cancer patients and the apparent protection afforded by agents that stimulate the immune system (discussed in the next section). However, the major argument against the validity of this theory is that protection by the immune system against tumor growth has only been observed with induced tumors. This has been shown in many experiments, one of which is the following. Spontaneous tumors were removed from an animal. Killed tumor cells were injected into a second animal, in order to generate an immune response. Then, live tumor cells were reinjected into the second animal. However, tumors formed, indicating that the second animal had not generated antitumor antibodies. Other types of experiments have supported the conclusion that some induced tumors cause an immune reaction, but this is rare for naturally occurring tumors. The reason for this difference is not known, but the following explanation is widely believed. Spontaneously arising tumors arise very slowly and pass through many biochemical and immunological changes before they can be detected. Experimentally induced tumors form very rapidly and are fairly uniform at the time of detection. When a long time has elapsed (as, for example, the time required to detect naturally occurring tumors), the cells have developed mechanisms for avoiding the immune response of the host; otherwise, they would not have survived to the point of detection.

Since spontaneously arising tumor cells usually do possess foreign or nonadult antigens, how do they avoid destruction by the immune system? One method is that described above, namely, that the cells continually change. In other words, as soon as antibodies have arisen that could destroy the tumor cells, the cells have changed and become resistant. A second mechanism is by saturating the immune system. Some tumors shed huge amounts of these antigens, and these cause a strong immune response. However, the production of the antigens occurs at such a high rate that the specific antibodies synthesized react mostly with these free antigens rather than with the antigens on the cell surface, and the specific killer cells have their receptors completely blocked by the circulating antigens. Third, some human malignant tumors release factors that suppress the immune system; presumably, this is a major cause of the weak immune response of patients with advanced cancer. Finally, some tumors cause the development of large populations of specific suppressor T cells that counteract the conversion of B cells to plasma cells, so production of specific antitumor antibody is weak. Details of how these four effects occur are not known.

The serum of patients with certain cancers such as melanoma and neuroblastoma contain protein factors that prevent T cells from attacking the cancer cells. These so-called "blocking" factors presumably coat the surfaces of the cancer cells, covering up tumor antigens, so the T cells cannot detect the antigens and cannot destroy the cancer cells (Figure 9-4). These blocking factors, which are poorly understood, may be antibodies made against tumor cell surface antigen. Instead of destroying the cancer cells, the antibody may bind to and cover the surface tumor antigens.

THE RATIONALE FOR IMMUNOTHERAPY

Even though immune surveillance may not be a major factor in the body's defense against cancer, a considerable body of evidence suggests that the immune system plays some role in cancer prevention. Thus, the possibility of preventing or curing cancer by immunotherapy has been examined in detail. An important observation that suggests that the immune system is at least one factor is that humans with genetic diseases that depress immune functions have a far greater frequency of cancer than normal people. A related observation is that patients that have been given immunosuppressive drugs to reduce rejection of transplanted organs (such as kidney transplant patients) also have a higher incidence of cancer than the normal population. Thus, various means of improving the strength of the immune response have been tried with animals and patients with small tumors and with humans with certain advanced cancers that are not responding to conventional treatment.

One method is injection of killed cells of Bacillus Calmette-Guerin, a nonpathogenic (attenuated) variant of a bacterium that causes tuberculosis. This bacterial suspension, which is called BCG vaccine, stimulates the immune system. Experiments with mice have shown that BCG given one week before injection of tumor cells often caused a substantial slowdown in tumor cell growth or sometimes complete tumor regression. Mice not receiving BCG vaccine before tumor cell injection exhibited extensive tumor growth, which eventually resulted in death of the animals. A variety of experiments have confirmed this observation but indicated that BCG vaccine is most effective if given before cancer cells appear in the organism, which makes it less useful for cancer patients. However, in a few cases promising results have been obtained in the treatment of people with advanced cancers. BCG vaccine has been observed to have striking effects on white blood cells, causing macrophages to become more active in destroying other cells and engulfing foreign substances. It also causes the macrophages to divide and synthesize more digestive enzymes. In tissue culture these activated macrophages will sometimes kill cancer cells, but not normal cells.

Another substance that may offer some promise in the immuno-therapy of cancer is called endotoxin, a substance isolated from the cell walls of certain classes (Gram-negative) of bacteria. If endotoxin is injected into animals with some types of tumors, hemorrhages develop in parts of the tumors and tumor regression occurs. Endotoxin seems to be most effective on established tumors. It is believed that endotoxin causes macrophages to release a tumor-killing factor. Recall Coley's work presented at the beginning of the chapter in which he injected cancer patients with killed bacteria, which resulted in tumor regression; these results may have been due to endotoxin in the walls of the bacterial inoculum.

A recent technological advance, the development of monoclonal antibodies, may provide a key to successful immunotherapy. This and other treatments will be described in Chapter 13.

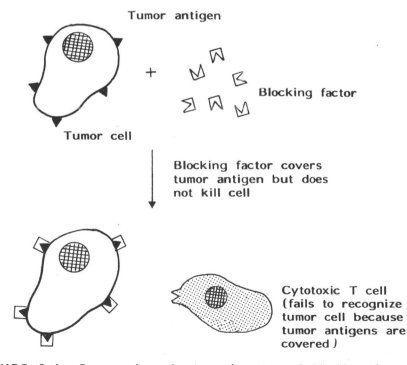

FIGURE 9-4   Presumed mechanism of action of blocking factors in protecting tumor cells against the immune system.

SPONTANEOUS REGRESSION OF CANCER

Spontaneous regression of cancer is the complete or partial disappearance of cancer not attributable to any treatment. Spontaneous regressions are rare, possibly as infrequent as 1 per 100,000 patients. A study of 176 cases recorded over a 70-year period suggested that removal of a carcinogen might account for some of the regressions. For example, in 10 bladder cancer patients both ureters had been diverted from the bladder to the bowel in preparation for removal of the bladder. Regression of the bladder cancer followed this preliminary surgery. It was suggested that a carcinogen in the urine might have been responsible for growth of the tumor, so when urine no longer accumulated in the bladder, the tumor shrank. Possibly, these patients had very effective immune systems that could eliminate the tumor cells once the carcinogen was removed.

Rejection of tumor cells by the immune system of the patient is a likely explanation for many spontaneous regressions. In one patient with malignant melanoma, regression followed a blood transfusion from a patient who previously had spontaneous regression of malignant melanoma. In another patient the regression followed a transfusion from a patient who had a 10-year cure after excision of a melanoma.

If indeed some type of immune reaction often destroys tumors when they are of microscopic size, spontaneous regression might simply be an example of a tumor that escaped the immune system long enough to grow to visible size but finally succumbed to attack by the system.

ADDITIONAL READINGS

Alberts, B. , D. Bray, J. Lewis, M. Raff, K. Roberts, and J.D. Watson. 1983. Molecular Biology of the Cell. Garland.

Burnett, F.M. 1971. "Immunological surveillance in neoplasia." Transplant. Rev., 7, 3.

Cole, W.H. 1974. "Spontaneous regression of cancer." CA., 24, 274.

Herberman, R.B. and H.T. Holden. 1978. "Natural cell-mediated immunity." Adv. Canc. Res., 27, 305.

Klein, G. 1973. "Tumor immunology." Transplant Proc., 5, 31.

Klein, G. 1975. "Immunological surveillance against neoplasia." Harvey Lectures, 69, 71.

Old, L. J. 1977. "Cancer immunology." Scient. Amer., 236, 62.

Ruddon, R.W. 1981. Cancer Biology. Chapter 7. Oxford.

Ting, C.C., S.C. Tasi, and M.J. Rogers. 1977. "Host control of tumor growth." Science, 197, 571.

10

Types of Tumors

So far, in this book we have considered the biology of tumor cells and how a tumor size arises. Now we begin to look at the finished product and examine the different kinds of tumors that form. We begin by comparing benign and malignant tumors and then look at the characteristics of some of the common types of malignant tumors.

BENIGN AND MALIGNANT TUMORS

A tumor is a tissue in which growth is uncontrolled. If the cells of the tumor remain differentiated and have the structure characteristic of their tissue of origin, the tumor is said to be benign. Such tumors usually grow very slowly as an expanding mass that is enclosed in a fibrous capsule. Some benign tumors stop growing and may even shrink. Benign tumors do not invade blood or lymph vessels and do not metastasize; they are harmful only in that they may put pressure on surrounding tissues. The term cancer is not applied to a benign tumor. To discover that a tumor is benign is a relief to both doctor and patient.

Malignant tumors (cancers) are usually (but not always) less differentiated than their tissue of origin. Malignant tumors are seldom encapsulated. Instead of being merely expansive, growth of malignant tumors is often invasive, infiltrating neighboring tissues, blood and lymph vessels, and body spaces. The capacity to metastasize is a major feature of malignant tumors. Note that a tumor is classified as malignant by the type of cells it contains; it need not have begun to invade nearby tissue or to metastasize to be called malignant.

CLASSIFICATION OF MALIGNANT TUMORS

Benign tumors typically are termed "omas" of specific tissues. In other words, the suffix "oma" is applied to a tissue to denote a benign tumor of that tissue, though some malignant tumors are sometimes inappropriately given this suffix. For example, glandular epithelial tissue is given the prefix "aden," so a benign tumor of glandular tissue is termed adenoma. A benign tumor of fibrous tissue is fibroma, while a benign tissue of cartilage is chondroma.

Malignant tumors are classified into two major groups, based on the tissue of origin. If a tumor arises in epithelial (surface) tissue, it is termed a carcinoma. These are the cancers of the internal and external surface linings of the body. The organ or specific tissue is often included in the name. Thus, skin cancer, or cancer of the epidermis, is epidermal carcinoma; cancer of the stomach lining is gastric carcinoma; cancer of the glands of the stomach is, more specifically, gastric adenocarcinoma ("adeno" refers to glandular tissue); and cancer of the adrenal cortex is termed adrenocortical carcinoma. The second major group, the sarcomas, includes cancers of mesodermal origin, that is, cancer of connective tissue, muscle, bone, blood and lymph vessels, fibrous tissue, fat, and cartilage. Special terms are again used to define the tissue of origin more precisely, namely, fibrosarcoma for cancer of fibrous connective tissue, liposarcoma for cancer of fat tissue, osteogenic sarcoma or osteosarcoma for bone cancer, leiomyosarcoma for cancer of the smooth muscle, and <u>rhabdomyosarcoma</u> for cancer of skeletal muscle.

The terminology used to describe various cancers is not as standardized as one might wish; there are numerous short terms used to denote certain malignant tumors. For example, the term <u>lymphoma</u> is often used instead of the more proper term, lymphosarcoma, to denote a certain type of cancer of the lymphoid tissue. <u>Leukemia</u> is cancer of the blood-forming tissue, the bone marrow. Instead of the term melanocarcinoma, the terms <u>melanoma</u> or malignant melanoma are used to identify cancers of the pigment-forming cells of the skin. Likewise the term <u>myeloma</u> is used to identify cancer of the antibody-forming plasma cells, instead of the more correct term, myelosarcoma. Cancer of the liver is usually termed <u>hepatoma</u> for hepatocarcinoma.

In addition to the rather bewildering list of terms given above, even more confusing are the cancers that are named after the person(s) who first characterized them. For example, the names Ewing's sarcoma (a form of bone cancer), Hodgkin's disease (a lymphosarcoma), and Wilms' tumor (a kidney cancer) do not tell anything about the tumor's origin or its malignancy. Although attempts at making the terminology of tumors as descriptive as possible are underway, it is unlikely that the nondescriptive terms that have been used for decades will disappear from usage.

We will now consider properties of individual tumors.

CANCER OF TISSUES AND ORGANS

In this section we describe the more important features of the most common cancers.

Lung

The most common form of lung cancer is that of the flat cells on the inner surface of the lung; this is called squamous cell carcinoma of the lung (squamous cells carcinoma of any tissue refers to growth from surface cells). These cancers usually form at the branches of the large bronchi. As the cancer grows, it invades the bronchi and lung tissue and metastasizes to the liver, bones, brain, and adrenal glands. Undifferentiated and <u>anaplastic</u> (without form) carcinomas of the lung are also rather common; the highly malignant oat cell carcinoma is of this type. Another major type of lung cancer is adenocarcinoma of the lung, which is a cancer of the glandular tissues in the lung surface linings. Cigarette smoking is the major cause of squamous cell and undifferentiated carcinomas of the lung. Metastasis occurs early in many lung cancers, and most patients with lung cancer cannot be cured, because present diagnostic techniques cannot identify these cancers at their early stages. Symptoms in lung cancer patients also usually appear relatively late in the history of the disease. It is likely that improvement in the early diagnosis of lung cancers will significantly improve the cure rates of this disease. This is one type of cancer that is clearly preventable by not smoking.

Cervix

Carcinoma of the cervix is one of the most carefully studied cancers, mainly because of the mass screening of women by the Pap test. It is first recognized by changes in the surface epithelium of the cervix, the so-called precancerous state. Later, the surface layers acquire a malignant appearance; this early stage, in which all cancer cells are on the surface is termed carcinoma in situ. Still later, the cancer begins to invade underlying connective tissue and extends into the vaginal wall, bladder, and rectum; this is true invasive carcinoma of the cervix, a stage in which metastasis is likely. Cervical cancer is curable when detected in the carcinoma in situ stage and when invasion has just begun. A Pap smear done regularly allows detection of this type of cancer at a sufficiently early stage, enormously increasing the likelihood of complete cure.

Skin

In Western societies skin cancer is the most common kind of cancer. The major types of skin cancer are basal cell carcinomas and squamous cell carcinomas. Basal cell carcinomas are the most common type and form from the lowest or basal layer of the skin. Growth is slow, and spreading seldom occurs. Basal cell carcinomas are often found in areas of the body exposed to the sun. They begin growth as shiny firm nodules in the skin (the most common form), an ulcerated crusted lesion, or a swollen scar. All of these forms enlarge and eventually ulcerate in the middle, after which they become covered with a scab or crust. If left untreated, these cancers may invade underlying tissues and metastasize, causing death either by hemorrhage or invasion of vital body tissues such as brain tissue. Infection may also be a cause of death.

Squamous cell carcinoma of the skin begins in the surface layer of the skin. These cancers usually grow slowly, but may begin to grow rapidly and metastasize to regional lymph nodes, ultimately leading to death. This cancer appears first as a red bump with a scaly or crusted surface, which finally becomes a firm red elevated nodule. The nodule ulcerates and sometimes reaches a diameter of one centimeter within a couple of weeks, invading the underlying tissue. Because this cancer may metastasize early in its development, it requires prompt attention and treatment. Both basal cell and squamous cell carcinoma have high cure rates when caught early.

The most malignant of the skin cancers is malignant melanoma (Figure 10-1). These cancers develop from cells that synthesize the pigment melanin in the skin. In rare cases, malignant melanomas may originate in a preexisting mole. For this reason, visible change in a mole should be promptly brought to the attention of a physician. However, most raised pigmented regions (moles, nevi, etc.) do not develop into cancers; melanomas usually form in normally colored skin. These cancers metastasize quickly and must be treated early for effective control. If not treated within a few weeks of the first noticeable enlargement, the prognosis (chance of cure) is quite poor. Melanomas occur most frequently in Caucasians, and although they usually occur in the 40-70 age group, they can also occur in younger individuals.

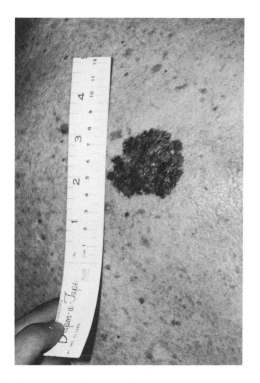

FIGURE 10-1 Malignant melanoma in a human. The cancer is always deeply pigmented and typically has an irregular border. Such a spot does not mean that cancer is necessarily present; diagnosis requires biopsy and microscopic examination. (Courtesy R.E. Saxton and D. Morton.)

Breast

The breast can be affected by a variety of cancers such as carcinoma of the ducts in the breast (duct carcinoma), carcinoma of the glandular epithelium of the breast (breast adenocarcinoma), and breast sarcomas and lymphomas. Adenocarcinoma of the breast usually presents itself as a hard, single nontender nodule. Metastasis occurs frequently by spread to regional lymph nodes. Most breast cancers can be detected by individual self-examination and can be controlled if detected sufficiently early that it has not spread to many lymph nodes. It remains the major cancer of women, but will probably be exceeded by lung cancer as the number of female smokers increases.

Liver

Most liver cancers are secondary, arising from metastasis; for these the prognosis is grim. The main primary tumor is a hepatocarcinoma (hepatoma); cells are either undifferentiated and embryonic in appearance or well differentiated, resembling normal bile duct lining. The differentiated type produces bile just as normal liver tissue does. There are many other types of liver cancers also. The incidence is quite high in the tropics, where it is believed to result from ingestion of aflatoxins from fungi growing in a moist environment. It is also associated with past cases of hepatitis. Patients with cirrhosis of the liver induced by excessive consumption of alcohol often develop primary liver cancer.

Colon-rectum

In Western societies this is the second-most common form of cancer. It is believed to be associated with diets with low contents of indigestible roughage. More than 80 percent of colon-rectum cancers are adenocarcinomas. Other types of colon-rectum cancer are far less frequent. When localized in the bowel or rectum, it is usually detected by the appearance of blood coating the stool. When higher up in the intestine, blood is not visible, but occult blood (trace amounts detectable only by enzymatic tests) is the presenting sign.

Bone

Bone cancer usually is first detected by persistent pains in joints or the extremities. Primary tumors are usually only found in children, whereas in adults bone tumors almost always arise by metastasis from other sites. Pain and swelling does not indicate malignancy, because bones are subject to a wide variety of benign tumors and cysts, and more often than not, the growth is not malignant. The most common malignancy is osteosarcoma, of which half are found at the ends of the bones of the leg near the knee. The patient is typically 10-20 years old. Ewing's sarcoma is a tumor of the so-called round cells of bone. There is considerable pain and swelling, and the tumor is generally quite extensive, including the entire shafts. The prognosis for bone cancer is not good unless the tumor is detected at a very early stage

Kidney

A variety of cancers of the kidney have been identified. Wilms' tumor (nephroblastoma) is an inherited kidney cancer of infants and children. This cancer is usually composed of tubular structures that are typical of the normal fetal kidney. However, the cells grow until a large mass has formed, then invades nearby tissues; it often metastasizes occurs early in the development of the cancer. Renal cell carcinoma is a common cancer in adults; it has a poor prognosis.

Prostate

Prostate cancer accounts for the majority of malignancies in males past the age of 65. It is usually a cancer of glandular tissue, an adenocarcinoma. It is recognized by a hard nodule that can be felt by the physician's finger. With routine physical examinations prostate cancer can be detected early enough that the cure rate is fairly high. However, it rapidly metastasizes to the pelvis and lower spine, after which the prognosis is poor.

Testicles

Testicular cancer is the most common cancer for males less than 30 years old. It arises from primordial germ cells. Depending on the particular cells, the tumors are called seminomas, teratomas, embryonal carcinoma, teratocarcinoma, and choriocarcinoma (which are listed in order of increasing malignancy). For unknown reasons, the frequency is 20-fold higher in males that had undescended testicles than in males in which descent was normal. Testicular cancer can be detected quite early by monthly self-examination as a hard nodule; when tumors are small, the prognosis is good.

Penis

Carcinoma of the penis is most common in uncircumsized men who practice poor personal hygeine. Presumably irritants accumulate under the foreskin, since the lesion invariably starts either on the underside of the foreskin or the covered portion of the penis. Partial surgical removal, leaving a substantial and usable stump, is quite successful; untreated it metastasizes to inguinal lymph nodes and then rapidly through the body.

Thyroid

Thyroid cancer usually presents itself as a symptomless hard lump in the lower part of the neck. It is not particularly malignant. Whereas numerous cancers have a slightly higher frequency in one sex or the other, the incidence of thyroid cancer is three times higher in women than in men (for unknown reasons). It is very frequently a consequence of early radiation exposure. Many years ago x rays were used to treated chronic tonsillitis, adenoiditis, acne, ringworm of the scalp, and enlarged thymus. The cancers usually develop about five years after radiation exposure, but patients free of disease after this interval are at increase risk for up to 40 years. The cure rate for early thyroid cancer is quite high, using a variety of different treatments, not necessarily using surgery.

Blood forming tissues

Leukemia is a cancer of the blood-forming tissues (bone marrow, spleen, lymph nodes, and thymus). There are a variety of leukemias, all of which involve overgrowth of normal blood-forming tissues by cancer cells derived from specific blood cell precursors, specifically, cells that develop into a variety of white cells. (There is a leukemia, which involves red cell precursors, but it is fairly rare.) The principal difference between leukemic and normal white cells is that leukemic cells remain immature and continue to divide.

The classification of leukemias is based mainly on the type of blood-forming precursor that is affected. The major types of leukemia are myeloid, monocytic, and lymphocytic. These are all cancers of the leukocytes or white blood cells. Myeloid cancer involves precursors to granulocytes (granular white cells responsible for engulfing bacteria and maintaining the integrity of the walls of blood vessels); monocytic leukemia involves monocytes (large motile lymphocytes responsible for engulfing cell and tissue debris); and lymphocytic leukemia is a cancer of lymphocytes. The terms acute and chronic are also used. In acute leukemia the cancer cells are primarily found in the tissue of origin (for example, granulocytes in the marrow and lymphocytes in lymph nodes).

For unknown reasons, different forms of leukemia prevail in distinct age groups. For example, acute lymphoblastic leukemia, in which the marrow becomes almost complete overgrown by primitive cells, is a disease of children less than 10 years old. In this disease there are huge numbers of dividing immature white cells. These cells do not function normally in protecting the host from infection, and infection is a frequent cause of death. Acute myeloblastic leukemia, in which a different type of primitive cell takes over the marrow, occurs mainly among people 25-50 years old. In late stages of this disease the cells invade the liver and spleen, causing severe anemia and loss of blood-clotting factors (with associated lethal internal bleeding). A variety of drugs are quite successful in the treatment of the early acute leukemias, especially in children. Chronic granulocytic leukemia occurs mostly in people 20-30 years of age. Primitive granuloctyes accumulate in the blood and colonize the marrow, spleen, and liver. Ultimately, almost all organs are affected. Patients seem remarkably healthy until near the end, when anemia, hemorrhaging, and fever become severe. Chronic lymphocytic leukemia prevails in the 50-70 age group. Primitive cells accumulate first in lymph nodes and other lymphoid tissue and finally replace the marrow. The ability to make antibodies decreases, and death usually occurs as a result of infection.

Myeloma is another cancer of white cells, this time the plasma cells, the differentiated white blood cells that produce circulating antibodies. The most common form is called multiple myeloma. In this disease, cancerous plasma cell foci are present in the bone marrow. These cells destroy normal marrow and the bone itself, giving the bone a punched out appearance in x-ray photographs. Mature-looking plasma cells are mixed together with the cancerous plasma cell precursors. The cancerous plasma cells produce great quantities of antibody, but the antibody is defective, and resistance to infection becomes very low. The cells also colonize the kidneys, causing total renal failure.

Lymphomas are cancers of another class of antibody-producing cells (the lymphatic and reticulendothelial systems). The most common type is Hodgkins's disease, primary cancer of the lymph nodes. It is characterized by swollen lymph nodes in the neck and upper part of chest, night sweats, and weight loss. Cancer cells gradually spread to lymph nodes and lymphatic tissue throughout the body. It is graded into four stages, depending on the location of affected nodes with respect to the primary tumor (for example, one node involved, multiple involvement, tumors on both sides of the diaphragm). At one time the prognosis for Hodgkin's disease was poor, but combinations of radiation treatment and chemotherapy are highly effective in stage-1 and stage-2 involvement. In non-Hodgkin's lymphoma the cervical and inguinal lymph nodes are common sites of the primary cancer. When detected, it has often spread to many parts of the body. Several anemia may develop due to bleeding in the digestive tract, and 20-40% of the patients develop leukemia.

This brief treatment of tumor types is simply intended to give the reader an overview of how tumors are classified. For more detailed description of any of the cancers, the reader is referred to any textbook on tumor pathology and histology, or to the Merck Manual.

ADDITIONAL READINGS

Cappell, D. F. 1958. Muir's Textbook of Pathology. Edward Arnold.

Merck Manual of Diagnosis and Therapy. 1982. 14th Ed. Merck, Sharpe, and Dohme.

Montgomery, G. L. 1965. Textbook of Pathology. Williams and Wilkins.

Ritchie, A. C. 1970. "The classification, morphology and behavior of tumors." In General Pathology, H. Florey, ed. Saunders, p. 668.

Robbins, S. L. 1974. Pathologic Basis of Disease. Saunders.

11

Epidemiology of Cancer

Epidemiology is the study of the natural history of disease. It includes examination of the incidence, distribution, environmental causes, and control of disease in population groupings. In this chapter, we shall summarize some of the data that have been accumulated through numerous epidemiological studies of cancer. Such data have revealed clues about the causes of cancer in specific groups of people; possibly, understanding the data will help to control certain cancers by identifying life styles of the groups that may be hazardous and can be modified. In this chapter we will present some of the results of epidemiological studies that indicate some of the cultural practices, habits, and occupations that may increase the incidence of particular cancers.

The first epidemiological data were obtained in 1775 when scrotal cancer in England was observed to be correlated with having been a chimney sweep as a child. This was the first example of an occupational cancer. In 1873 it was noted in Germany that workers in the tar industry frequently developed cancer on their hands and arms. In time, other industrial agents, such as dyes, were implicated in causing cancer in workers. Now most epidemiological data on cancer are obtained on a fairly large scale, often by government and cancer research organizations. The most important data of the past 20 years are the subject of this chapter.

CANCER AND AGE

A most significant feature of cancer incidence is that the frequency of almost all cancers increases with age (Figure 11-1 and Table 11-1). For example, data compiled by the United States Public Health Service show that the death rate from colon cancer increases more than 1000-fold between the ages of 30 and 80. In the age group 20-30 the incidence is one death from colon cancer per million people per

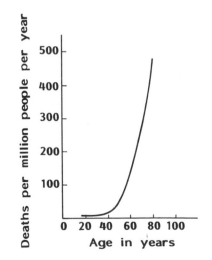

FIGURE 11-1   Death rate from colon cancer in relation to age.

year, while in the age range 60-80 there are >1000 deaths per million people per year. From such data various hypotheses have been expounded that attempt to account for the dramatic increase of many cancers with age. The most widely accepted theory is that both the initiation and promotion steps required for transformation occur at low frequency, so a long time is required before both events have occurred. This reasonable idea has not been proved rigorously though. Table 11-1 also shows a sex dependence of cancer incidence at all ages; the reason is unknown.

IS CANCER INFECTIOUS?

The possibility that cancer may be infectious has been raised by laymen, cancer epidemiologists, and experimental cancer researchers. Examination of the distribution of cancers in certain communities has been suggestive. Clusters of cancer cases have been identified that occur among individuals related by contact. Hodgkin's disease and leukemia are two types of cancer that has exhibited such clustering. However, careful statistical analysis shows that these clusters could easily be the result of chance rather than infection. On the other hand, there is some evidence that cancer of the cervix can be spread by sexual contact, because it is most common in women with several sexual contacts, especially when young. Circumstantial evidence implicates herpes viruses, which are easily transmitted by sexual contact, in the development of some cervical cancers; however, no statement can be made that herpes is the cause of these cancers. Burkitt's lymphoma, discussed in Chapters 6 and 10, is clearly associated with Epstein-Barr virus. However, even though the virus clearly is transmitted between individuals, there is no evidence that the cancer is also transmitted directly, because infection by the virus is insufficient to develop the cancer. Recall that a large fraction of the Caucasian population of North America has been infected with this virus, yet Burkitt's lymphoma is unheard of in North America. One possible reason also shows up in epidemiological data: namely, that more than half of the people with this disease had malaria as children; if exposure to malaria is a prerequisite to acquiring the lymphoma, the disease would not be found in North America, where malaria does not occur.

That certain cancers of animals are infectious is quite clear, and these are all virally induced. For example, viruses appear to be an important factor in causing leukemia in cats, chickens, and mice. Whole flocks of chickens can be decimated by a leukemia-like condition called Marek's disease, which is transmitted by a herpes virus and can be prevented if the chickens are vaccinated with viral material. In these forms of animal cancers viral infection must be sufficient to cause the cancer, or else the promotion step must occur very frequently in these animals. Once feline leukemia was well documented, the question of transmission of leukemia from diseased cats to their owners obviously became important. However, the incidence of leukemia among cat owners is no higher than among those who do not own cats, so such transmission must be considered to be exceedingly unlikely. In fact, there is no correlation between any virally induced

TABLE 11-1 Mortality for the five leading cancer sites by age group and sex (U.S., 1977)

Under 15 Male	Under 15 Female	15–34 Male	15–34 Female	35–54 Male	35–54 Female	55–74 Male	55–74 Female	75+ Male	75+ Female
Leukemia 633	Leukemia 422	Leukemia 755	Breast 623	Lung 10,110	Breast 8,348	Lung 44,112	Breast 17,341	Lung 14,060	Colon & Rectum 11,953
Brain and Nervous System 414	Brain and Nervous System 302	Brain and Nervous System 474	Leukemia 553	Colon & Rectum 2,434	Lung 4,528	Colon & Rectum 13,504	Lung 13,045	Prostate 11,645	Breast 8,166
Bone 58	Bone 47	Testis 423	Brain and Nervous System 316	Pancreas 1,307	Colon & Rectum 2,283	Prostate 8,851	Colon & Rectum 12,190	Colon & Rectum 8,811	Lung 4,341
Connective Tissue 50	Connective Tissue 46	Hodgkin's Disease 352	Uterus 303	Brain and Nervous System 1,200	Uterus 2,093	Pancreas 6,378	Ovary 6,000	Pancreas 3,205	Pancreas 3,778
Lympho- and Reticulosarcoma 49	Kidney 35	Skin 254	Hodgkin's Disease 235	Leukemia 1,046	Ovary 2,063	Stomach 4,652	Uterus 5,573	Bladder 3,121	Uterus 2,970

Source: Vital Statistics of the United States, 1977. Cited in *Cancer Facts and Figures*. New York: American Cancer Society, 1980.

cancer in animals and cancer in humans, indicating that human cancer cannot be contracted by exposure to diseased animals.

EPIDEMIOLOGICAL STUDIES OF PARTICULAR HUMAN CANCERS

Epidemiology has helped us obtain important information about factors involved in a variety of specific cancers. Some of these cancers and the relevant information will be described in the sections of this unit.

Lung Cancer

Lung cancer afflicts >100,000 Americans today. Studies of the habits of more than a million people indicated in the 1960s that about 80 percent of those affected were cigarette smokers, and that the incidence of lung cancer is six times greater among smokers than nonsmokers. Recent studies over a 12-year period by the American Cancer Society implicate cigarettes even more strongly by showing that the probability of cancer correlates with the composition of the cigarettes used. For example, the lung cancer death rates among individuals who smoked low-tar and low-nicotine cigarettes was 26 percent lower than the rates for high tar-nicotine cigarette smokers. Furthermore, the lung cancer rate is reduced among smokers who stopped smoking, though it still is very high compared to the rate for those who never smoked. These studies make it reasonable to expect that a major reduction in smoking could lead to the near elimination of one of the most deadly of all cancers.

Lung cancer death rates are also high among workers in radioactive ore mines and in workers that contact asbestos, chromium, and nickel. Smokers who also work in the asbestos or radon industry have an even higher incidence of lung cancer than the industrial nonsmokers or smokers alone. It seems clear that taking carcinogens into the lungs is asking for an early death.

Stomach Cancer

Studies of the incidence of stomach cancer in different communities have yielded quite striking information. For example, stomach cancer death rates are high in Japan, Iceland, Chile, Austria, Finland, Central Europe, and the Soviet Union, but low in the United States, New Zealand, Canada, Israel, and Australia (Table 11-2). Catholics and Protestants have higher rates than Jews. People with blood-type A and people in low socioeconomic groups have higher rates, as do individuals with pernicious anemia and achlorohydria (no acid is produced in the stomach).

A clue to possible causes of this type of cancer comes from studies that show that stomach cancer death rates drop significantly among Japanese who have immigrated to the United States (Table 11-3). The drop is most pronounced in first generation Japanese-Americans. This information has suggested that perhaps a change of diet is responsible for the reduced stomach cancer rate. Individuals having a high risk

TABLE 11-2   Regional differences in cancer incidence

Cancer	Highest incidence	Lowest incidence
Men		
Skin	Queensland	Bombay
Esophagus	Northeast Iran	Nigeria
Lung	Great Britain	Nigeria
Stomach	Japan	Uganda
Liver	Mozambique	Norway
Prostate	U.S. (Blacks)	Japan
Colon	Connecticut, U.S.	Nigeria
Oral cavity	India	Denmark
Rectum	Denmark	Nigeria
Bladder	Connecticut, U.S.	Japan
Women		
Cervix	Colombia	Israel (Jews)
Breast	Connecticut	Uganda

of stomach cancer generally have diets that are low in fresh fruits and vegetables and high in starches such as rice, potatoes, and bread. Thus, it is possible that the drop in stomach cancer rates in Japanese-Americans is due at least in part to a change in diet with, for example, a reduction in rice consumption and increase in use of fresh fruits and vegetables. At one time, it was thought that the high rate of stomach cancer in Japan was caused by aflatoxin (a potent carcinogen) in soy sauce. A fair amount of recent evidence has ruled out this possibility and implicates the high consumption of salted fish and many preserved foods, which are rich in nitrosamines; the role of salted fish has not been proved though. High peat content in soil may also play some role in increasing stomach cancer risk in certain countries. High concentrations of nitrates in the water supplies in countries such as Chile may increase the risk of stomach cancer. However, other data in the United States do not suggest that stomach cancer is associated with these nitrates.

Colon-Rectum Cancer

Colon-rectum cancer is very common in the United States and approaches lung cancer in accounting for >100,000 new cases each year. These forms of cancer have higher mortality rates in North America (especially in the East), most of Western Europe, New Zealand, and Australia than in the Caribbean, Central America, the Eastern Mediterranean, Southeast Asia, Japan, and Sub-Saharan Africa. Unlike stomach cancer, Jews and high socioeconomic groups have higher colon cancer death rates than Protestants, Catholics, and lower socioeconomic groups, possibly because the higher socioeconomic groups simply live longer and hence have a higher probability of contracting the condition.

Examination of the diets of these various groups suggests that a diet low in fiber and high in simple sugars probably increases the risk of colon and rectal cancer. Colon cancer may also be related to dietary fat intake. The incidence of colon cancer is higher among workers in the asbestos (probably due to ingestion of asbestos fibers) and rubber industries, and among machinists (ingestion of metal dust?) and footwear workers than in the general population. The incidence of colon cancer is lower in agricultural workers and wood processors. Individuals with a history of ulcerative colitis, colon polyps or familial polyposis of the colon, diverticulitis, or appendicitis have increased risk of colon-rectal cancer.

Esophageal Cancer

Esophageal cancer in whites in the United States is associated with the use of alcohol plus tobacco. Studies on blacks in the United States with this form of cancer have not yet been reported. In an area of South Africa, esophageal cancer is very common and associated with molybdenum deficiency. In Curacao, a high incidence of esophageal cancer is associated with high consumption of medicinal teas made from certain plants that contain potent carcinogens.

Bladder Cancer

Bladder cancer is high among workers in industries that deal with carcinogens such as aniline dyes, aromatic amines, benzidine, and 2-napthylamine. Boiler makers, plumbers, structural metal workers, and welders also have increased bladder cancer rates, which may be caused by metal found to be excreted in the urine. Possibly metal particles serve as irritants. Bladder cancer is high in New Jersey, rural New York and New England, and in urban areas around the Great Lakes where large numbers of individuals work in the chemical industry, instrumentation manufacture, lumber, and industries manufacturing items of wood, stone, clay, and glass. Higher bladder cancer rates are found in England, Scotland, and parts of South America, whereas they are low in Asia, Ireland, parts of the Caribbean, Norway and Sweden. Bladder cancer death rates are higher in female Protestants,

TABLE 11-3 Cancer deaths and immigration: death rates of Japanese males per one California white male (age adjusted)

Cancer	In Japan	Immigrants	Sons of immigrants
Stomach	6.5	4.6	3.0
Liver	3.7	2.1	2.2
Colon	0.2	0.8	0.9
Prostate	0.1	0.5	1.0

low or middle socioeconomic groups, and in individuals who are not married. Increased risk of bladder cancer is found in patients with a history of chronic bladder infections or kidney stones. Cigarette smokers also have increased risk for developing bladder cancer, but no correlation has been established between bladder cancer risk and alcohol consumption. There is also no connection with the total amount of liquid consumed per day (that is, over or underuse of the bladder)

Cancer of the Cervix or Uterus

Individuals who have had frequent and early sexual intercourse, many broken marriages, and early marriages have increased risk of cervical cancer. Women whose sexual partners are uncircumcised and who also do not practice personal cleanliness are more prone to cervical cancer. Some workers believe that cervical cancer may, in some cases, be related to infection with herpes virus, because individuals with cervical cancer often had past histories of genital herpes infection. Cervical cancer is more frequent in women who have a very large number of children and who are in low socioeconomic groups. It is rare in virginal and Jewish women. Cervical cancer death rates are high in parts of Africa, Asia, and Latin America, but low in North America, Europe, Australia, and New Zealand.

Breast Cancer

The breast is the leading site of cancer in women (Table 11-1) and is the leading cause of death in the 40-44 age group. Breast cancer mortality is higher in upper socioeconomic groups and among Jewish women. The following factors predispose toward breast cancer: unmarried, one or two children, over age 35, infertile, first pregnancy past age 25, menarche before age 12, 30 or more years of menses, a history of breast cystic disease, and mothers or sisters with breast cancer. The following characteristics are associated with a rate of breast cancer less than average: continuously married, fertile, <30 years of menses, receiving pelvic irradiation during ages 40-44 years, three or more children, under age 35, first pregnancy under age 25, menarche at age 15 or older, and having had hysterectomies, especially those combined with bilateral removal of ovaries before age 40. Breast cancer death rates are low in Japan, Soviet Union, Far Eastern Asia, the Caribbean, and Africa.

Prostate Cancer

Death rates from prostate cancer are higher in white married men 54-74 years of age than in single men of the same age group. Jews from all socioeconomic groups have lower death rates than Protestants and Catholics. High prostate cancer death rates occur in the United States, Canada, Belgium, France, Scandinavia, Switzerland, Australia, and New Zealand. Individuals immigrating to the United States from Japan and Poland have higher prostate mortality rates than native Japanese and Poles. Prostate cancer death rates are low in most of Africa, Asia, and Latin America. In the U.S. mainland and Hawaii, prostate cancer death rates were found to be lower in non-blacks and non-Caucasians than in Caucasians and blacks. Prostate cancer incidence in American blacks is the highest in the world (Table 11-2).

Leukemia

Death rates for leukemia (all types except chronic lymphocytic leukemia) are high among survivors of the atomic bomb blasts in Japan, among patients irradiated for ankylosing spondylitis, and among radiologists. These data point to excessive exposure to radiation as a significant risk factor for all types of leukemia except chronic lymphocytic leukemia. Children with leukemia are more likely to be those from older mothers than from younger mothers, and leukemia mortality rates are usually higher in Jews than in Protestants or Catholics. Leukemia rates are also high in operating-room personnel exposed to anesthetics and in rubber solvent workers such as those working with benzene.

Skin Cancer

Skin cancer is most frequently found in blond Caucasians with fair skin and is less common in blacks. It is more common in men than in women, possibly because men, who are less concerned that the appearance of their skin than women, are more likely to allow their skin to come in contact with chemicals and harsh irritants. It seldom occurs in children, simply indicating that repeated exposure to carcinogens over a long period of time is necessary for the cancer to develop. The high frequency of skin cancer among outdoor workers, compulsive sun tanners, and people who live in the sun belts clearly indicates that overexposure to the sun is a primary (if not the major) cause of skin cancer. The propensity for fair-skinned individuals to develop the cancer is likely to be a result of their inability to synthesize sufficient quantitities of protective pigment. Industrial carcinogens, irritants, and radioactive materials also can cause skin cancer, which has been inferred from studies of the incidence of skin cancers in individuals repeatedly exposed to such agents.

HOW EPIDEMIOLOGICAL DATA CAN BE USED

Epidemiological studies have served to identify some important cancer-causing agents, such as tobacco products, certain industrial chemicals, and radiation. These conclusions are unambiguous. Major risk factors have been summarized in Table 11-4. However, when examining risk factors such as age groups, race, westernized versus nonwesternized countries, socioeconomic groups, religions, and so forth, the information does not lead to immediate conclusions. Rather, it provides stepping stones for further investigation. The general approach is to examine the life styles and habits of these groups and to seek common features. They are, however, not easy to see, especially when the factor is socioeconomic group or religion.

An example of the approach can been seen in an attempt to understand why gastrointestinal cancer is more prevalent in affluent

TABLE 11-4   Major risk factors, based on epidemiological data

Colon-rectum	Breast
History of rectal polyps Rectal polyps in family History of ulcerative colitis Blood in stool Over age 40	History of breast cancer Close relatives with this cancer Over 35; especially over 50 No children First child after 30
Lung	Skin
Heavy smoker past age 50 Started smoking < age 15 Smoker worked near asbestos	Excessive exposure to sun Fair complexion Worked with coal tars
Uterine-endometrial	Oral
Late menopause (after 55) Diabetic, high blood pressure, and overweight Age >50	Heavy smoker or drinker Poor oral hygeine
	Ovary
Uterine-cervical	Close relatives with this cancer Age >50

Frequent sex in early teens
  or with many partners
Low socioeconomic group
Poor care during or following
  pregnancy
	Never had children

	Stomach
Prostate	Close relatives with this cancer Diet heavy in smoked, pickled, or salted foods
Age >60	

westernized societies. It seems reasonable to predict that cancers of the digestive tract will be related to materials that pass through the tract, namely, the food we eat. By examining the diets of individuals with, for example, colon cancer, factors such as diet low in fiber, high in beef, and high in fat appear repeatedly. With this sort of information, researchers have designed experiments utilizing different components of beef, different fats, etc., to determine specifically which of these factors are truly carcinogenic in animals. Sometimes an educated guess can be made. For instance, the rate of passage of material through the intestine has been compared for diets low in fiber and high in fiber, and it has been observed that passage is more rapid with high-fiber diets. On this basis, it has been hypothesized that the value of high dietary fiber is to decrease the residence time of carcinogens in the large intestine by moving the material through the colon rapidly.

ADDITIONAL READINGS

American Cancer Society. 1977. "Lung cancer and smoking." Cancer Facts and Figures. American Cancer Society, pp. 19-20.

American Cancer Society. 1980. Cancer Facts and Figures. American Cancer Society.

Fraumeni, J.F. 1975. Persons at High Risk of Cancer. Academic Press.

Grufferman, S. 1977. "Clustering and aggregation of exposures in Hodgkin's disease." Cancer, 39, 1829.

Higginson, J. 1969. "Present trends in cancer epidemiology." Canad. Cancer Conf., 8, 40.

High Background Radiation Research Group. 1980. "Health survey in high background radiation areas in China." Science, 209, 877.

Lilienfeld, A.M., Levin, M.L., and Kessler, I.I. 1972. Cancer in the United States. Harvard University Press.

Silverberg, E., and Holleb, A. I. 1974. "Cancer statistics, 1974. Worldwide epidemiology. CA—A Journal for Clinicians 24, 2.

12

Diagnosis of Cancer

At present, early diagnosis of cancer offers the most hope for effective treatment and cure. It is likely that new methods in the early diagnosis of cancer will be at least as important as new methods of treatment, and past history suggests that this is the case. For example, cervical cancer, if diagnosed early, is usually curable. The Pap test has done a great deal in identifying early cases of this disease, and it is likely that the observed increased cure rates for cervical cancer can be attributed in large part to early diagnosis. We noted earlier in the text that once cancer cells have spread away from the primary tumor, the chance for cure is dramatically decreased. Early diagnosis simply increases the chances of identifying and treating a cancer before it has spread.

Two factors limit early detection: that state of the present technology and the attitude of many individuals. Both of these problems lead to treatment failure. The technical problem is simply that most modern methods of diagnosis usually cannot detect an internal cancer until it is about one centimeter in diameter. Such a cancer contains approximately one billion cells. Some lung cancers or breast cancers may require ten years or more to reach this size, by which time the cancer has already begun to spread. If left untreated, many individuals with such cancers would not live very long after spread has occurred, so by the time many cancers are diagnosed, the life of the patient is nearly over. Improved methods (still under development) of early diagnosis will dramatically affect the cure rate of many types of cancer. The second problem is a psychological one: some individuals do not make themselves available for diagnosis until late in the history of the cancer (they do not see a physician, because they are "afraid of what the doctor will find").

We begin this chapter by describing some standard methods of cancer diagnosis and then examine a few promising new approaches.

STANDARD METHODS OF CANCER DIAGNOSIS

The individual, rather than a physician, is usually best able to detect symptoms of an abnormal condition in the body (Table 12-1). Therefore, it is often the patient who detects a lump, an abnormal skin condition, a change in bowel habits, or respiratory or swallowing problems and brings it to the attention of a physician. However, significant observations can be made in the annual or biennial physical examination, the first topic of this section.

Routine Physical Examination

The routine physical examination is designed to seek out a variety of potential health problems. In the course of such an exam a physician or physician's assistant will always looks for signs of cancer. The routine cancer screening usually includes the following examinations:

1. Visual skin examination and palpation (pressing with the fingers or hand) of areas in the skin to check for lumps, sores, swellings, or discolorations. Change in the appearance of a wart or mole can be a symptom of malignant melanoma of the skin,

which is one of the more difficult cancers to treat if not detected exceedingly early. If any region of the skin is unusual, a small piece of the tissue is excised and then examined with a microscope (that is, a biopsy is done).

2. <u>Palpation of lymph nodes</u> in the neck, and palpation of the larynx and thyroid for enlargement, tenderness, and immobility.

3. <u>Inspection of mouth</u>, tongue, palates, cheeks, floor of mouth, larynx, pharynx, and tonsil area. The patient is asked to swallow, and signs of obstruction are sought.

4. <u>Lung examination</u> via stethoscope, X ray, and/or microscopic examination of sputum or mucus that is coughed up; the latter sometimes reveals the presence of cancer cells.

5. <u>Breasts are inspected and palpated.</u> The breast is examined with the woman's arms lowered and raised. Irregular contours, skin dimpling, and other abnormalities may be a symptom of unusual tissue growth. The lymph nodes in the neck are palpated for enlargement, and the breasts are palpated in a rotary fashion while the woman is seated, lying, and with arms behind her head. The nipples are squeezed for evidence of discharge, and the lymph nodes in the armpits are felt. Detection of breast lumps or lymph node enlargement may indicate a need for further evaluation. A mammogram (a type of low-dose x-ray diagnostic technique) is sometimes recommended for high-risk patients such as those with a family history of breast cancer. Routine use of mammography for low-risk patients is controversial because x rays themselves increase the risk of cancer.

6. <u>Vaginal and cervical examinations</u> are conducted, and a cervical smear (Pap test) is taken for microscopic examination of cells. The Pap test reveals if the lining of the uterine cervix consists of normal cells or cells with varying degrees of abnormal structure. A sample of uterine lining can also be taken for microscopic examination in those patients at high risk of developing endometrial cancer (cancer of the inner lining of the uterus).

TABLE 12-1   Key diagnostic warning signals for cancer

CANCER'S 7 WARNING SIGNALS

Change in bowel or bladder habits
A sore that does not heal.
Unusual bleeding or discharge
Thickening or lump in breast or elsewhere
Indigestion or difficulty in swallowing
Obvious change in a wart or mole
Nagging cough or hoarseness.

If YOU have a warning signal, see your doctor!

Source: American Cancer Society.

7. Rectum and colon examinations are accomplished by finger
    examination of the rectum and tests for invisible blood (occult
    blood) in the stool. When blood is seen and no tissue masses
    can be felt, direct visual examination of the rectum and lower
    colon may be carried out by proctoscopy or sigmoidoscopy. In
    males the prostate gland is also palpated through the rectal
    wall.

Numerous other diagnostic tests are used if there is reason for
suspicion. These include x-ray examination of the digestive tract,
brain, and other organs of the body, as well as urine and blood
tests.

Biopsy

The ultimate test for cancer is a microscopic examination of cells to
determine if the cells are normal or abnormal in structure or growth
pattern. Cells are obtained in three ways: from biopsy (removal of
small pieces of tissue excised from a suspicious area), from smears
(as in the Pap test), and from fluids such as sputum, blood, or
lymph.

A biopsy sample may be obtained in a variety of ways. For
example, a sample may be obtained simply by inserting a needle in
the tissue and withdrawing a small number of cells (a needle biopsy).
Tissue from the lung or stomach is often obtained by insertion of a
hollow tube into the organ. The tube contains fiber optics, which
enables the physician to see exactly where the tube is going, and
forceps may be passed through the tube to excise a small piece of
tissue. (The instrument used for lung examination is called a flexible
bronchoscope, for it can be passed into branches of the bronchi.) In
some cases, local or general anesthesia is required to obtain biopsy
samples. When tumors, which may or may not be malignant, are
definitely evident, the biopsy specimen may be taken early in the
course of internal (major) surgery, and quickly frozen and sectioned
in order that microscopic examination of the tissue can be made during
the operation. In this way, the surgeon can learn about the nature
of the tumor without delay, and if cancer is indicated, the surgeon
can remove the tumor immediately.

Biopsy material is normally examined by a pathologist or a well-
trained technician. Various features of the tissue are examined to
determine whether the tissue is malignant. Usually, tissue that is
malignant is anaplastic, which means without form; that is, the cells
are not arranged in the way expected of the tissue of origin. It is
often undifferentiated, made up of cells that lack many of the
characteristics of the normal tissue types from which the cancer was
derived. A cancer of glandular tissue will less and less resemble the
normal glandular organization as the cancer becomes more malignant.
The cells may not form distinctly shaped glands, but instead may
form irregularly shaped structures, or columns of cells; in extreme
cases, the cells lack all attachment to neighboring cells and appear
to be growing without any organization. Cells in malignant cancers
often have abnormally shaped nuclei containing several deeply staining

bodies called nucleoli. Such cells also often have larger nuclei than normal cells. These visual features, plus intense staining by certain dyes, are often reliable indicators that the cells are cancer cells. If cells of this type are observed in the biopsy tissue to have invaded blood vessels, lymph vessels, or normal tissues, malignancy is assured. On the other hand, if the tumors is surrounded by a fibrous capsule, and if the tumor cells closely resemble cells of the normal surrounding tissue, often highly differentiated like the tissue of origin, the tumor is undoubtedly benign. In such tumors invasion of surrounding tissue, blood or lymph vessels is not observed. Finally in a benign tumor no cellular abnormalities or unusual nuclei are seen. In summary, the classification of tumors with respect to malignancy is based on a variety of criteria that include the pattern of cells in the tissue and the characteristic appearance of the cells themselves.

In an interesting study done several years ago, laboratory technicians who examine biopsies were asked to describe in words the difference between normal tissue and cancerous tissue. Surprisingly, a variety of quite varied visual criteria were described; however, when they were presented with numerous tissue samples, the technicians agreed almost completely on the classification.

Smears and fluid tests

Instead of using a tissue section to determine the nature of a tumor, a scraping or smear can be taken. A smear differs from a biopsy not only in the way the cells are obtained, but also that the smear consists of mostly individual cells and small clumps, so tissue organization cannot be determined. Therefore, the pathologist is somewhat handicapped, because judgment must be based solely on cellular characteristics such as the appearance of the nuclei and cytoplasm mentioned above. An additional problem is that the sample usually contains many fewer cells than that obtained by a biopsy, and cancers cells might be missed. In the case of vaginal smears, the diagnosis based on such smears is 85-98 percent correct, with false positives being rare and false negatives accounting for the errors. Even though smears are more limited than biopsies, nonetheless pathologists become quite skilled, and smears are exceedingly important diagnostic tools.

A test related to a smear in that a fairly small number of individual cells is sampled is what might be called a fluid test. Some examples are sputum (obtained by coughing up mucus), bronchial washings, nipple discharges, and liquids from the bile and pancreatic ducts. The cells are stained and examined in much the same way as for a smear.

More will be said about smears and fluid tests in the next section when we examine how specific cancers are diagnosed.

SYMPTOMS AND DIAGNOSIS OF SPECIFIC CANCERS

In this section we present some of the information and tests that are used in diagnosing particular types of cancer. This summary is not intended to be exhaustive or a rigorous medical analysis but is instead designed to sample the ways by which cancer diagnoses are established.

Cervical and Uterine Cancer

The Pap test, the most commonly performed smear tests, is a valuable procedure for screening for cancer or the uterus and cervix. A smear is taken from the upper vagina, which contains secretions from the vagina, cervix, and lining of the uterus, and the cells are examined by microscopy. The smears are classified in the following way:

Class I: Normal.

Class II: Probably normal, but possibly with slightly atypical cells.

Class III: Doubtful that it is normal due to the presence of clearly atypical cells; probably precancerous or cancerous.

Class IV: Probably cancer. Cells are very atypical, overly large, and with abnormal shape. Nuclei are enlarged and stain abnormally.

Class V: Unmistakable cancer. Cells are clearly even more abnormal than Class IV smear.

If abnormal cells are seen, tissue is taken for biopsy to determine whether the cells are precancerous or cancer, for the treatment would depend on the diagnosis. The cervix, because of its accessibility, has been exceedingly well studied, and the various transitions from normalcy to invasive cancer are well known. A brief description follows.

A normal lining of the cervix is characterized by a regular layer of columnar cells that is surrounded by a multilayered vaginal lining. Slight abnormalities such as thickenings of the surface lining are common. A condition termed dysplasia, which can be considered as precancerous, is characterized by an abnormal arrangement and size of cells in the lining. Dividing cells, usually found in only the deepest layers of cervical area, are scattered through most of the layers. Dysplasia may develop into a localized tumor called carcinoma in situ; in this condition, cells are less differentiated and more abnormal, but the cancer is localized in the surface layers of the cervical lining, and the cells have not invaded the underlying connective tissue. In a later stage, the abnormal epithelial cells invade the underlying tissues, and true invasive cancer is present. Such cells can penetrate blood and lymph vessels and spread to distant parts of the body. Determination of dysplasia, carcinoma in situ, and invasive cancer is based in large part upon the organization of cells in a tissue, rather than just the appearance of individual cells, so accurate diagnosis depends upon procuring an adequate piece of tissue.

Intermenstrual and postmenopausal bleeding is a common symptom of cancer of the endometrium (uterine lining). Vaginal discharge, bleeding, and itching suggest the possibility of cancer of the vulva. Premalignant whitish plaquelike or ulcerated lesions often precede cancer of the vulva. Vaginal discharge, spotting, pain during intercourse, groin masses, and urinary abnormalities are symptoms of possible vaginal cancer.

Lung Cancer

In the early stages of lung cancer, when it is more curable, there are often no symptoms. The lucky patient will have the cancer detected in a routine chest x ray or sputum sample. The most common early symptom of lung cancer, particularly cancer of bronchi, is a persistent cough, unaccompanied by symptoms of a virus infection. In later stages, there is blood in the sputum, weight loss, chest pain, shortness of breath, or pneumonia. X-ray examination can detect lung cancers, but often, if symptoms are present, the diagnosis is too late, having been made only after spread has already occurred. This is the primary cause of the dismal statistics on lung cancer survival. Aberrant x rays in the symptomatic or asymptomatic patient are usually followed by direct visual examination of the interior of the lung by a flexible fiber-optic bronchoscope. With this instrument, sampling of lung tissue is possible without the need of opening the chest or lung. Microscopic analysis of the sputum for evidence of cancer cells are promising methods for early detection of the disease, though many false negatives are obtained.

Colon and Rectum

A change in bowel habits is the most common symptom of cancers of the colon and rectum. Diarrhea, bleeding, constipation, or lower abdominal pains persisting for more than several days should be reason for further evaluation by a physician. Cancers of the rectum and colon can often be diagnosed early with present techniques. A finger probe can often detect a rectal tumor and a proctosigmoidoscope can be used to detect a tumor several inches into the colon. X ray diagnostic technique and fiberoptic colonoscopes are also useful in revealing colon cancers. The colonoscope can penetrate more than a foot into the colon and also enables the physician to remove a small biopsy sample. A common form of x-ray diagnosis is made by filling the colon with a liquid barium solution; the solution is opaque to x rays and all tissue appears as more transparent material. Abnormal thickening of the wall of the intestine and small tumors can be seen on the x-ray film by this technique.

Prostate Cancer

Both benign and malignant tumors are not uncommon in the prostate of elderly men. Early prostate cancer seldom presents any symptoms. However, as the tumor increases in size, urinary problems begin to appear. These include interrupted or weak urine flow, difficulty in urinating or in stopping urine flow, increased frequency of urination, blood traces in the urine, pain or burning during urination, and pain in the lower back, pelvis, or upper thigh. Fortunately, most prostate enlargements are not cancerous. Cancer can occasionally be detected by the presence of cancer cells in urine or seminal fluid, but normally a biopsy is needed for diagnosis. A needle biopsy may be sufficient.

Cancer of Mouth, Throat, and Nasal Regions

Cancers of the lip, oral cavity, and tongue often appear first as ulcers that fail to heal within a few weeks. Bleeding without cause may also be a symptom. Cancer of the salivary glands may present itself as enlarged glands. Cancer of the nasal passages may be associated with bloody nasal discharge, obstruction in breathing, neurological symptoms, or the presence of masses. Persistent hoarseness is a key important early symptom of cancer of the larynx (voicebox), while pain on swallowing is often associated with throat cancer. Many diligent dentists include a cancer exam as part of a checkup of the general condition of the mouth. Careful palpation of all tissues of the mouth, tongue, and cheek can often show a thickening of the tissue, which may be an early cancer. Visual observation of all tissues of the mouth by the dentist or physician may show characteristic red, white, or darkly colored patches that may be precancerous. Biopsy of suspicious tissue is essential

Thyroid Cancer

A lump in the thyroid gland is often the first symptom of thyroid cancer. Hoarseness and difficulty in swallowing may also be present. Two techniques, biopsy and thyroid scans, are utilized for diagnosis. In a thyroid scan the patient ingests a short-lived radioactive iodine isotope. Iodine is rapidly localized in the thyroid, since it is a component of the the thyroid hormone, thyroxin. All normal regions of the thyroid gland become radioactive as thyroxin is made. However, the tumor tissue is mostly undifferentiated, does not synthesize thyroxin, and hence doe not become radioactive. The distribution of radioactivity throughout the thyroid gland is then determined by a variety of imaging techniques. Presence of a nonradioactive region is highly significant and cause for biopsy or surgical excision.

Cancer of the Esophagus

Difficulty in swallowing solid foods is often a prime symptom of cancer of the esophagus. Fiber optical instruments are used for direct viewing of the interior of the esophagus. X-ray visualization of the esophagus, and microscopic examination of esophageal washings to detect cancer cells are also common diagnostic procedures. Unfortunately, by the time esophageal cancer is symptomatic, metastasis has usually occurred.

Stomach Cancer

Stomach cancer (gastric cancer) often first becomes evident by long-term upper abdominal discomfort, loss of appetite, or weight loss. Upper gastrointestinal x-ray examination (upper GI series) is an accurate diagnostic method for stomach cancer, for large tumors can be seen in the x-ray photographs. Examination for occult blood in the stool (blood produced in the stomach but no longer evident as free blood), analysis of stomach acid, microscopic examination of gastric washings for cancer cells, and fiber-optical examination of the stomach are also standard procedures for establishing a diagnosis.

Cancers of the Liver, Gallbladder, and Pancreas

Cancers of the liver, gallbladder, and pancreas are difficult to detect, and diagnosis is seldom achieved in the early stages of these cancers. Liver scans (using particular radiochemicals as in the diagnosis of thyroid cancer) and biopsies establish the presence of liver cancer. Weakness, vague upper abdominal pain or discomfort, anemia, jaundice, or respiratory distress may also be present in liver cancer cases, especially since metastasis is frequent. Cancer of the gallbladder is usually not diagnosed until the gallbladder has been removed following symptoms characteristic of acute inflammation of the gallbladder. In the case of pancreatic cancer, abdominal pain not related to digestive function and persistent weight loss often present themselves. Occult blood in the stools, jaundice, and clay-colored stools may also occur. Pancreatic cancer is invariably detected well after metastasis has occurred, and hence the prognosis is exceedingly poor.

Cancer of the Kidney

Kidney cancer in adults is another disease that is usually without symptoms until late in the development of the cancer. The ultimate symptoms include blood in the urine, back pain, and a palpable mass, though on occasion only fever, malaise, weight loss, and weakness are present. Wilms' tumor is a kidney cancer of children that usually presents itself with abdominal swelling, loss of appetite, and general discomfort. Various x-ray techniques, blood, and urine analysis are used to diagnose kidney cancers. Ingestion of radioactive salts of technetium, which localize in normal kidney tissue, followed by radioactive scans, can often detect small tumors as nonradioactive masses.

Bladder Cancer

Blood in the urine is the most common symptom of bladder cancer. Lower abdominal pain, pus in urine, frequent and urgent urination are also often present. X-ray examination of the bladder following ingestion of radioopaque compounds (cystoscopy) and biopsy are used to confirm diagnosis.

Cancer of the Testes and Penis

Cancer of the testes is commonly detected as a painless hard region in one testis followed by a general hardening and enlargement of the whole organ; a vague sensation of heaviness and aching in and around the scrotum may also be noticed by the patient. Cancer of the penis may appear as a sore that does not heal in a reasonable time, bleeding during erection or coitus, itching, or discharge. The most common tumor sites are the corolla and the underside of the foreskin. Cancer of the penis is seldom seen in circumcised men.

Breast Cancer

A lump in the breast is the most common symptom of breast cancer. Skin or nipple retraction is also an important symptom. Occasionally symptoms such as erosion of the nipple surface, or watery or bloody discharge present themselves early in the disease. Breast swelling, redness, ulceration of the skin, and lymph node enlargements are some of the signs of advanced breast cancer. X rays are usually taken to learn more about a suspicious lump, because they can detect spotty calcifications and increased tissue density characteristic of breast cancer. Routine x-ray photography (mammography) may be done with high-risk patients or those with symptoms that suggest breast cancer. Since women are subject to a variety of nonmalignant growths in the breast, a biopsy is essential for accurate diagnosis. Biopsies are sometimes performed by withdrawing material through a large bore syringe, which can be inserted into the tumor (needle biopsy), or by a small incision.

Cancer of the Ovary

Early ovarian cancer is often symptomless. Advanced ovarian cancer may present symptoms such as weight loss, occasional vaginal bleeding, painful or increased frequency of urination, and constipation. A feeling of abdominal heaviness may be present, caused by fluid accumulation in the abdominal cavity. This fluid, called ascites, may contain a large number of cancer cells. Routine pelvic examinations and immediate evaluation of any ovarian enlargement are crucial to diagnosing ovarian cancer before it is too advanced for successful treatment.

Bone Cancer

Persistent pain in a bone is the most common symptom of bone cancer, though it may be associated with a variety of nonmalignant cysts. The bone pain often follows a bruise, fall, or trauma, but does not go away. An evident bony growth is sometimes, but not usually, a symptom. X-ray examination is usually used to look for tumors. If radioactive phosphate is administered, the phosphate is localized in rapidly growing tissue such as bone tumors; radioactive scans can usually detect regions of intense radioactivity. Conclusive diagnosis requires biopsy, which may be obtained by a needle or minor surgical techniques.

Cancer of the Central Nervous System

Early symptoms of cancers of the brain and spinal cord generally depend on the region of the brain or spinal cord in which the tumor is located. The symptoms are initially simply a result of pressure by the tumor. Personality changes, such as bizarre behavior and irritability, are associated with tumors of the frontal lobe of the brain.

Headache, dizziness, and difficulty in walking are associated with tumors in the cerebellum. Vision changes and convulsive seizures may also be associated with some brain tumors. In general, a brain tumor is suspected whenever there are slowly progressive signs of dysfunction. A variety of neurological examinations are made when brain tumors are suspected: for example, visual and hearing tests, x rays of the chest (for sources of metastasis) and of the cranium, electroencephalography (for changes in the electrical properties of various parts of the brain), and CAT scans (described later in the chapter). Brain tumors are very often benign, but even these are hazardous because of the consequences of intercranial pressure. Tumors of the spine are much less common than brain tumors. The symptoms are again those of pressure, usually on a nerve root. Analysis of the pattern of loss of function usually indicates where the pressure is, and x rays of the area indicate whether the pressure is a result of a nerve tumor, bone tumor, or simple arthritic changes, the latter being the most common.

Lymphomas and Multiple Myeloma

Lymphomas are cancers of the lymphoid tissues in the body and usually present themselves as lymph node enlargement. Other symptoms such as weight loss, malaise, and excessive night sweating may be present. Lymph node biopsy is required for accurate diagnosis. Lymphoma does not always start in lymph nodes but may begin in lymphoid tissue of the spleen, bone marrow, liver, lungs, or other organs of the body. Multiple myeloma is a cancer that originates in the bone marrow and results from excessive proliferation of cells that synthesize antibody (plasma cells). Pain or weakness of bones are sometimes indicative of the disease. Accurate diagnosis of multiple myeloma is based on urine analysis for a particular type of proteins (Bence-Jones proteins) produced by the aberrant plasma cells. In addition, x-ray evaluation of the bones of patients with multiple myeloma shows characteristic empty lesions throughout the bone.

Leukemia

The major sign of leukemia is a combination of long-term fatigue, weakness, and low-grade fever. These symptoms are so common for many viral infections, such as colds, that they are unfortunately often not followed up. Later stages of leukemia are characterized by severe weakness, pain in bones or joints, and enlargement of lymph nodes, liver, and spleen. In very late stages bleeding without apparent cause occurs. Symptoms of acute leukemias appear suddenly and progress rapidly. Chronic leukemias, on the other hand, often go undetected for years and are usually detected by routine blood examination. Two major diagnostic tests are used to identify leukemia. A blood test is used to determine the number and types of white blood cells; in leukemia the white cell count is very high and many immature cells are seen. The definitive test is a bone marrow biopsy; bone marrow is generally removed by puncture of the pelvic bone, and an analysis of the white cells in this tissue is made. The bone marrow of individuals with acute lymphocytic leukemia is characterized by replacement of normal marrow with lymphoblasts (immature lymphocytes) and more mature lymphocytes. Other types of leukemia are characterized by the presence of other cell types. Blood tests are usually not sufficient, because in many patients with early leukemia the marrow contains many cancer cells, yet the blood is normal. Furthermore, in some cases of children with acute lymphocytic leukemia, the white blood cell count may fluctuate widely, sometimes very high and sometimes normal, or even be reduced.

NEW TECHNIQUES IN CANCER DIAGNOSIS

The goal of cancer diagnosis is to detect the tumor as early as possible, preferably before it has reached the invasive stage. A variety of new techniques, many requiring significant advances in engineering and computer technology, are helping physicians achieve this goal. A few of the more commonly used techniques will be described

Computerized axial tomography (CAT) is a recently developed technique that overcomes the major disadvantage of standard x-ray photography, namely, the inability to see soft tissue clearly. X rays are excellent for bone, for small amounts of calcified tissue, and for large amounts of soft tissue, but fail almost completely to detect small portions of soft tissue. In the CAT technique a narrow beam of x rays passes through the body, and the intensity is detected by a bank of fluorescent crystals. The beam moves, sweeping across the area of the body to be imaged, and small differences in the intensities of the transmitted beam are analyzed by a computer. Many sweeps of the beam are made, each one looking through a narrow section of the body. The computer processes the intensities in successive layers of the body and constructs a three-dimensional picture of the area. The picture is displayed on a television screen or can be transferred to photographic film. The result is that one can accurately determine the shape, size, and location of small regions of the body; for cancer detection, CAT scans enable very small tumors to be detected and precisely located. CAT scans are particular valuable in examining fairly inaccessible parts of the body, such as the brain. The technique is sufficiently sensitive that cancers can be visualized that escape detection by other more standard techniques. The single disadvantage of CAT is the extraordinary expense of the machine, and the fact that a scan takes so much longer than a standard x ray that the number of patients that can be examined in one day is quite small compared to the number who can be x-rayed.

Ultrasound (the use of high frequency sound waves, also called diagnostic ultrasonography) can be used instead of x rays to locate tumors deep inside the body. In this completely harmless technique pulses of high frequency sound waves are passed through tissue and echoes are detected. The amount of sound transmitted and reflected is determined by the density of the tissue. By using suitable sound detectors and computer analysis a three-dimensional photograph of small regions of the body can be obtained. This method supplements the information obtained by CAT scans. By a variation of the technique regions in which the tissue density changes periodically, for example, pulsing arteries and arterioles, can be detected. In this way, ultrasonic techniques can be used to determined whether a tumor contains large blood vessels. Ultrasound is sufficiently harmless that it has been used to detect the position of a fetus before birth. In cancer treatment it is often used with patients undergoing radiation therapy for precise location of the tumor.

Certain tumors produce particular embryonic antigens, such as carcinoembryonic antigen (CEA) and alpha-fetoprotein (AFP), and blood tests have been developed to detect these antigens. Large tumors often release large amounts of CEA into the circulation; smaller tumors release tiny amounts, but with the development of sensitive immunological techniques such as the radioimmunoassay, CEA can be detected in minute amounts. Measurement of CEA has been used to diagnose early cancer of the colon and rectum, since about 90% of the patients have detectable CEA in the blood. However, the presence of CEA does not mean that a cancer is definitely present, for several reasons. First, the amount of CEA found is significant, and CEA is produced in association with certainly noncancerous conditions, for example, inflammation of the intestine. In a study of more than 10,000 individuals 97% of healthy nonsmoking adults had CEA in their blood at a concentration below 2.5 nanograms (ng) per milliliter. About 72% of patients with colon and rectal cancer, 76% of patients with lung cancer, and 91% of patients with pancreatic cancer had CEA in their blood at higher concentrations. However, individuals with nonmalignant disease sometimes showed elevated CEA concentrations. For example, 71% of patients with alcoholic liver cirrhosis and 57% of patients with emphysema had elevated CEA levels. Interestingly, 19% of smokers with no clinical signs of any of these diseases also had elevated CEA levels; possibly, these people will develop palpable cancer in the next decade.

Alpha-fetoprotein is not normally found in adults, except for those with hepatitis or with hepatoma (a type of liver cancer) or teratocarcinomas of the testis. If hepatitis can be ruled out, the presence of the antigen can be taken as evidence for cancer; this is valuable, since the test is exceedingly sensitive and will detect very early tumors.

Test for these antigens are also useful in determining whether treatment has been successful. For example, if a tumor making CEA is surgically removed, the concentration of CEA in the blood usually returns to normal levels rapidly. If the concentration does not decrease or goes up again, some cancer cells probably remain and are growing. Such an increase or lack of decrease would indicate the need for chemotherapy or radiation treatment, which would otherwise not be done.

SUMMARY

Late diagnosis of cancer often means treatment failure; early diagnosis often means cure. Therefore, diagnostic techniques take on a central role in the effective management of cancer. Those cancers that presently have a poor prognosis are usually those in which early diagnosis is seldom achieved. Development and utilization of new diagnostic tools, such as CAT scans and immunological tests to detect tumor antigens, will in all likelihood improve the cure rates for cancers that previously were detected relatively late in their development.

ADDITIONAL READINGS

A Cancer Source Book for Nurses. 1975. American Cancer Society.

Baker, R.R., Marsh, B.R., Frost, J.K., Stitik, F.P., Carter, D., and Lee, J.M. 1974. "The detection and treatment of early lung cancer." Ann. Surgery. May.

Brett, G.Z. 1969. "Earlier diagnosis and survival in lung cancer." Brit. Med. J., 4, 260.

Davies, D.F. 1966. "A review of detection methods for the early diagnosis of lung cancer." J. Chron. Disease, 19, 819.

Dunphy, J.E., and Way, L.W., eds. 1975. Current Surgical Diagnosis and Treatment. 2nd ed. Lange Medical Publications.

Eddy, D.M. 1980. "Guidelines for the cancer-related checkup: recommendations and rationale." CA, 30, 208.

Eddy, D.M. 1980. Screening for Cancer: Theory, Analysis, and Design. Prentice-Hall.

Knepp, M.A., and Chatton, M.V., eds. 1976. Current Medical Diagnosis and Treatment. Lange Medical Publications.

Leffall, L.D. Early Diagnosis of Colorectal Cancer. Amer. Canc. Soc. Prof. Educ. Publications.

Morra, M., and Potts, E. 1980. Choices: Realistic Alternatives in Cancer Treatment. Avon.

Robbins, S.L. 1976. Pathologic Basis of Disease. Saunders.

Strax, P. 1976. "Control of breast cancer through mass screening." J. Amer. Med. Assoc., 235, 1600.

Various publications are available from the American Cancer Society, local cancer societies, and clinics and hospitals about self-examination for breast and testicular cancer and about the general question of self-examination.

13

Treatments for Cancer

When cancer is diagnosed early before spreading has occurred, many cancers are curable. Furthermore, even when not curable, cancer is always treatable, substantially increasing the life of the patient. In this chapter, we will examine the three standard forms of cancer treatment: surgery, chemotherapy, and radiation therapy and will also describe a few experimental treatments that are not yet in widespread use.

SURGERY

For many cancers the treatment of choice is surgery, for surgery can, in favorable cases, completely remove a cancer. If the cancer is totally removed before the cancer has spread, permanent cure may result. Even when complete removal is not possible, if the cancer has not spread, the number of cancer cells can be reduced sufficiently that the natural defenses of the body can sometimes destroy the remaining cells. Alternatively, chemotherapy and/or radiation treatment can be used to complete the job. In any case, reducing the size of a tumor, even one that has spread, often prolongs life.

A variety of surgical techniques, some which do not even utilize cutting of tissue, are used in treating cancer. A localized cancer that has not spread is usually removed by simple excision of the tumor along with a small amount of the surrounding tissue. This technique is used for most noninvasive basal cell carcinomas and some squamous cell (surface) carcinomas. If tumor cells have spread to regional lymph nodes, these are also removed. In some cases, nearby lymph nodes are removed to be on the safe side; they are sectioned and examined by a pathologist. If no cancer cells are present, nothing has been lost; however, if cancer cells are seen, other nodes further along the lymphatic pathway are usually examined.

A technique is considered to be surgical if tissue is destroyed or removed; cutting is unnecessary. Several techniques of this sort are used in treating cancer. One of these is cryosurgery, the use of liquid nitrogen probes to freeze the tumor; the freezing kills the cells without the possibility of spreading any cells around by the operation of cutting. This technique is used in treating some cancers of the brain, prostate, and oral cavity. Another technique is electrosurgery, which effectively burns the tumor by touching it with electrical terminals; it is effective with some cancers of the rectum, skin, and oral cavity. Chemosurgery utilizes caustic pastes and is effective in treating skin cancers. These pastes burn or erode away the tumor and must be carefully applied to achieve successful results. Frozen sections of the tissue under treatment with such pastes are made to determine if the cancerous area and a margin of surrounding tissue have been removed.

Surgery is also used as a means of preventing cancer. A variety of premalignant lesions, such as radiation ulcers, villous adenomas of the colon, facial keratoses (rough raised bumps), and leukoplakias (white regions) of mucous membranes often become malignant if not excised. Carcinoma of the penis and cervical carcinomas (in females) are greatly reduced in frequency with circumcision during infancy of the male partner. A variety of benign polyps of the colon, cervix, and stomach are often surgically removed to reduce the possible risk of developing malignancy.

Surgery is also useful in removing advanced cancer that is blocking a duct or organ, even though such surgery may not remove the entire cancer. Such surgery is worthwhile if it eases symptoms such as pain, bleeding, effects of gastrointestinal blockage, anemia, vomiting, or anxiety. Although the patient may not be cured by such treatment, quality and length of life may be significantly improved.

Greatest success from surgery occurs when the primary tumor is removed before spreading has occurred, as we have said. However, even after spreading, cures can be achieved by surgical removal of a metastatic secondary tumor if only one such tumor is present and if the tumor is a slow-growing type.

The prognosis for cancer patients with tumors that are treatable by surgery depends on a variety of factors, principally the size and growth rate of the tumor and whether invasion has begun. Tumor size is important, because as the tumor increases in size, the probability of metastasis is increased. For example, the prognosis for melanomas less than 2 cm in diameter is statistically much better than for larger ones. The growth rate of the tumor is also significant. Generally, patients with undifferentiated rapidly dividing cancers have a poorer prognosis than those with well differentiated, slow-growing tumors. Whether invasion has occurred is extremely important. Cancers that invade surrounding tissues as they enlarge are more dangerous than those that enlarge without spread of peripheral cell groups into surrounding tissues. Cancer cell invasion into blood vessels usually means a poorer prognosis because of the increased possibility that such a tumor has spread. As more nearby lymph nodes show cancer cells, the outcome becomes more dismal, because this is an indication that the cancer has spread through the lymphatic system.

Some factors that may affect prognosis after surgical excision of a cancer are poorly understood. These include the patient's ability to mount an effective immune response against small numbers of remaining cancer cells, and the general physical condition, emotional condition, and age of the patient. These factors probably play a major role in the patient's ability to deal with various potential complications of the surgery and the cancer itself.

Surgical removal of various parts of the body often have profound emotional effects on cancer patients, and more and more is being done to alleviate these difficulties. Artificial limbs, esophageal speech and mechanical speech techniques, plastic surgery, and breast prostheses (rebuilt breasts) help many patients to return to a normal life style. Teams of rehabilitation professionals work with the patient and family to help the patient recover physically and emotionally from extensive cancer surgery.

RADIATION THERAPY

For many cancers radiation therapy is the treatment of choice. We have previously mentioned that radiation can cause cancer, probably by damaging chromosomes in cells, but radiation can also effectively kill cells. It is this killing power and the ability of radiotherapists to concentrate the killing power in very localized regions that form the basis for the very successful use of radiotherapy in treating some cancers.

Various radiations, such as x rays, gamma rays, electrons, protons, and neutrons, are used in radiotherapy. X rays are generated by bombarding a metal target in a vacuum tube by high speed electrons; the bombarded metal atoms produce the x rays (Figure 13-1). Gamma rays, which are more energetic, are emitted by certain radioactive isotopes; the most common ones in use in cancer therapy are cobalt-60 and radium. New methods of radiotherapy involve use of high energy neutron beams and beams of other atomic particles. The choice of radiation depends both on what is available at a particular hospital or cancer center and the degree to which the radiation must be localized.

Radiation therapy is carried out in four basic ways (Figure 13-2). (1) The entire body is exposed to radiation from radioisotopes or x-ray units. This is called whole-body radiation and is used primarily in cases of widely disseminated cancer, such as leukemia or advanced metastases. (2) Radiation is beamed into the patient from a tiny opening in a radiotherapy unit. The beam is carefully localized either by visual alignment or with computer-controlled focusing, so that the patient receives much of the killing power at the cancer site and not in normal tissues. This is the most common type of radiotherapy (Figure 13-3). (3) Radioactive isotopes are placed in the cancer itself

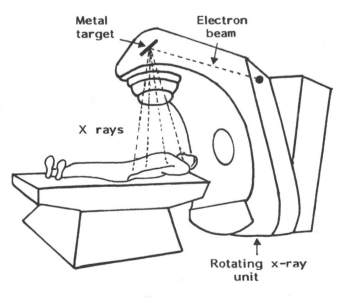

FIGURE 13-1 A schematic diagram of a therapeutic x-ray machine. An electron beam strikes a metal target, which then produces x rays. By use of appropriate metal apertures the x rays can be formed into a narrow beam (not shown).

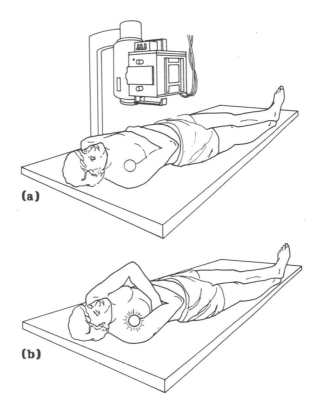

FIGURE 13-2 Two kinds of radiotherapy. (a) A small x-ray unit. (b) Radioisotope implant.

with needles, capsules, or other such devices that bring the radiation directly into the tumor (Figure 13-4). This is often done following surgical excision of a localized tumor to ensure that any residual cells are destroyed. (4) Radioisotopes that localize only in particular tissue are ingested. An example is radioactive iodine, which is localized exclusively in thyroid tissue and can be used to treat thyroid cancer.

Radiation kills all cells by causing biochemical changes that interfere with the ability of the cell to continue dividing. The basis of radiation therapy is that cells committed to division are more sensitive than resting cells, since both condensed chromosomes and the mitotic apparatus itself is particular sensitive to radiation. However, death of normal cells certainly occurs as a result of the radiation. What is important is to choose a dose of radiation that will kill many cancer cells (that is, the dividing cells) and produce minimal damage to the normal cells. Figure 13-5 shows a graph relating shrinkage of tumors ("tumor lethality') and death of normal tissue with various doses. It can be seen that a dose can be administered (e.g., 5000 to 6000 rads) that causes death of many tumor cells but only of a small fraction of the normal cells. However, unless all of the tumor cells are killed, the technique will not be successful. With

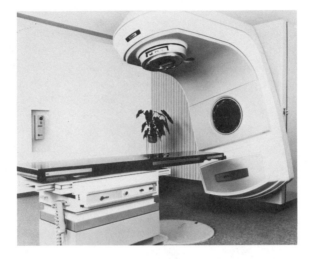

FIGURE 13-3 A large x-ray machine. These large units are usually made so the beam can be rotated around the patient, thereby minimizing damage to healthy tissue. Compare to Figure 13-1. (Courtesy of Varian Assoc.)

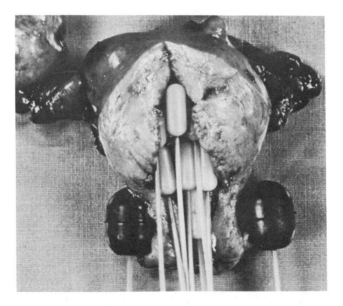

FIGURE 13-4 A uterus specimen showing how implants of radioactive materials would be applied to the internal organ. (Courtesy of Nuclear Associates.)

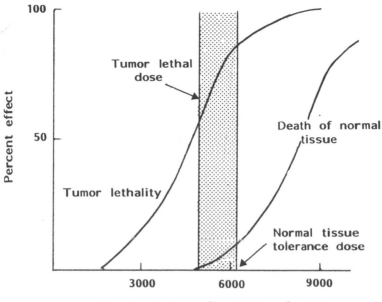

FIGURE 13-5 A graph relating death of various cells (as percent effect) versus radiation dose, for tumors and for normal cells. The stippled region is a dose that causes extensive killing of tumor cells with minimal killing of normal cells.

a single dose, most of the nondividing cells will not be killed. However, by allowing time to elapse (days) after delivering the initial dose, many of the cancer cells that were not dividing at the time of the initial dose will be in the division phase, and much of the normal tissue will have had time for repair. Giving a second dose at this time will cause more of the cancer cells to be killed, again with minimal damage to normal tissue. With repeated cycles of irradiation follows by a time interval of a few days, ultimately all of the cancer cells can be killed (at least in the irradiated region). At this time, a period of a few months will surely allow complete repair of all normal tissue.

One factor acts against the use of radiation. The chemistry of radiation damage is quite complicated and includes production of a large number of reactive intermediates that diffuse through tissues and cells and damage both the bases and the sugar-phosphate strands of DNA. The production of both types of intermediates require the presence of molecular oxygen. In some types of tumors the cancer cells have lower amounts of oxygen than do normal cells, either because of an inadequate blood supply or because of particular biochemical features of the cells. This has the effect that more radiation is required to kill these cells, and for a given degree of killing, more normal cells may be killed than in the tumors (these considerations do not apply to well-vascularized tumors). This problem can however be circumvented by using so-called densely ionizing radiation, such as pi mesons and ions accelerated by cyclotrons and similar machines. When passing through matter, these particles produce, without needing oxygen, a great deal of molecular damage; furthermore, the damage tends to occur directly in DNA. Neutron beams are also quite useful with tumors of this sort, because neutron-mediated damage also does not need oxygen. When using these radiations there is still a certain amount of oxygen-dependent damage that occurs in the normal tissue. This can be reduced by treating the tumor area with chemicals (radiation protectors) that decrease production of oxygen-dependent intermediates (peroxides) in oxygenated normal cells. Other compounds, called radiation sensitizers, can also increase radiation killing power in cancer cells by increasing the production of certain intermediates in oxygen-poor cells.

Whenever cells are destroyed, new cells are formed by cell division to replace the dead cells. Thus, killing tumor cells may stimulate rapid growth of new tumor cells. For this reason, radiation is most effective with the slow-growing tumors, because these cells do not respond to death of neighboring cells by extensive proliferation. On the other hand, normal cells in the surrounding healthy tissue quickly replace dead cells. In summary, in slow-growing tumors cancer cells are less likely than normal cells to repopulate an area that has been destroyed, so irradiation is a valuable treatment.

In addition to rapidly growing cancers other types of cancer can not always be treated successfully with radiation, for reasons that are sometimes obscure. Those that do respond well to radiation therapy are the following:

1. Cervical cancer. Radiation is administered by an x-ray or cobalt-gamma machine or by an implant of a radioisotope such as radium directly into the cervix. Implants are frequently done after removal of a cancerous ovary or uterus. Often, following routine hysterectomies small foci of cancer cells are seen in the tissue. A cervical radium implant is then done to kill any cells that may have left the tiny primary tumor and penetrated the cervix.

2. Early cancer of the vocal cords. Surgical intervention for cancer of the larynx almost invariably will cause loss of the voice, certainly if the larynx or the vocal cords must be removed. However, with radiation treatment the vocal cords are left intact and the voice is preserved fairly well, often without any change. Therefore, radiation therapy is the treatment of choice for many early laryngeal cancers, and a high cure rate (about 85 percent) is achieved.

3. Cancer of the tongue. Radiation is administered by radium needle implants and sometimes additionally with x rays or gamma rays. The cure rate is high and the tongue does not have to be removed.

4. Hodgkin's disease. This is a cancer of the lymph nodes. If only a small number of nodes are involved, x irradiation of

diseased lymph nodes (and the surrounding regions) combined with preventative radiotherapy of normal lymph nodes is often curative. Other types of lymphoma can also be cured with radiation therapy, especially if diagnosed early.

5. Germ cell cancers. Seminoma, a testicular cancer, is often cured by combination of surgery, and radiation therapy. Ovarian dysgerminomas are also treated successfully with localized radiotherapy, without the need to remove the ovaries.

6. Ewing's sarcoma. Ewing's sarcoma, a usually fatal form of bone cancer of children and young adults, is treatable by new methods of intensive radiotherapy of the cancer combined with drug therapy. Recently reported results suggest that such treatment may, in some cases, be totally curative.

7. Brain cancer. Brain tumors are frequently inoperable, and generally radiotherapy is the treatment of choice. Medulloblastoma, a brain cancer that is most often found in children, is quite effectively treated with radiotherapy; in fact, it can only be cured with radiation. Densely ionizing radiation is often used with brain cancer because the radiation can be deposited in a highly localized region, minimizing damage to surrounding brain tissue.

8. Skin cancer. Many skin cancers are cured with radiotherapy, thereby avoiding the extensive tissue damage and scarring that may result from surgical excisions.

9. Thyroid cancer. Thyroid cancer that has spread to other parts of the body can be treated by having the patient drink a radioactive iodine "cocktail." Thyroid cancer cells as well as normal thyroid tissue take up iodine. The cancerous thyroid gland is removed surgically, and the patient is given a hormone that stimulates growth of thyroid cells. The only thyroid cells present are the thyroid cancer cells, which may be anywhere in the body, so there is a specific stimulation of the cancer cells. Short after giving the hormones, the radioactive iodine cocktail is given, and thyroid cancer cells that have spread take up the radioactive iodine. Amounts of the radiochemical are given that are sufficient to kill any cell that has taken up the material.

10. Other cancers. Cancers such as Wilms' tumor (a childhood cancer of the kidney), bladder cancer, retinoblastoma of the eye, and neuroblastoma (a cancer of the nervous system usually occurring during childhood) all can be effectively treated with radiation therapy or radiotherapy combined with chemotherapy and/or surgery.

Although radiotherapy is exceedingly useful, it is not without problems, the principal one being side effects of various consequence. These side effects are sometimes related to destruction of nearby healthy tissue, but are more often a result of inflammation of the specific organ or tissue being treated. For example, diarrhea frequently follows irradiation of any pelvic tumor because of irritation of the colon and rectum. Nausea is associated with many radiation treatments, in particular, those for breast cancer and Hodgkin's disease. In general, the more extensive is the radiation and the higher the dose, the more like nausea is to occur. Recently, it has been found that treatment with marijuana significantly decreases the nausea and other radiation-associated malaise. Sore throat frequently occurs in patients being irradiated in the head and neck regions. Since cells that manufacture hair are normally dividing, irradiation of the head region often causes loss of hair. Unless the doses are very high, the hair returns several months after the treatment. Mild skin burn results if a large radiation dose is given. In general, the side effects of radiation can usually be easily controlled by medication, improvement in diet, and/or reduction of heavy smoking and/or drinking.

The use of beams of heavy ions (produced by cyclotrons or other accelerators) minimizes many of the side effects, especially with deep-seated tumors. These particles enter tissue and, when first penetrating, lose very little energy. As they penetrate more deeply, the rate of loss of energy increases, until they finally lose almost all of their energy over a distance of less than 0.01 mm. This has the beneficial effect of highly localized damage with very little damage to normal tissue; in fact, the energy of the particles can be chosen so that all of the damage occurs within the tumor. Negative pi mesons are also useful in this respect. These particles, which are produced by bombarding a beryllium target with high energy protons, pass quickly through normal tissue with relatively little damage to the tissue. Their energy can be chosen to that they slow down in the tumor, where they are captured by carbon, nitrogen, and oxygen atoms. This capture phenomenon results in the localized production of x rays and a variety of particles including protons, alpha particles, and neutrons. Thus, localized radiation within the tumor is caused by negative pi meson capture.

It has been estimated that radiotherapy can potentially cure 60 percent of all cancers. Perfection of newer techniques and increased availability of these procedures may result in a significant improvement in the cure rate of some cancers that today are not responding well to conventional forms of treatment.

CHEMOTHERAPY

Chemotherapy is the treatment of cancer with drugs. It is very effective in some forms of cancer. A major success story is with certain forms of childhood leukemia, which not too long ago was considered incurable. Today, utilization of combinations of drugs has led to long term remissions (apparent absence of the disease) and probable cures of this and other cancers. In the early 1970s the number of cures resulting from chemotherapy was <10,000. By 1980 improved drugs increased this number to >40,000.

Chemotherapy is based on the fact that certain drugs (antitumor drugs) are more active against cells in the cell cycle than cells in the G_0 phase (which are considered to have left the cell cycle). Death results from aberrant preparation for DNA synthesis, production of defective DNA, and aberrant mitosis. Some tumors are cured by the drugs, because a large fraction of their cells (perhaps even the majority) are, at any particular moment, making DNA and dividing. Thus, the principle of chemotherapy is no different from that of radiation therapy; only the means of producing the damage differ. Tumors are most curable by chemotherapy when they are young and the fraction of the cells in active growth is very high. However, just as in radiation therapy, repeated doses are given to allow cells in resistant stages of the cell cycle to enter the sensitive phases. In older and larger tumors, the growth fraction is quite low, and chemotherapy alone is usually not effective.

Unfortunately, no drugs have yet been found that kill all cancer cells and no normal cells. Furthermore, there are few cancers that can be cured permanently by a single dose of a drug or even by repeated doses of the same drug. Instead, treatment schedules must be devised that result in maximum cancer cell kill with minimum kill of normal cells. Such schedules often involve the use of more than one drug. Since some cells in cancers tend to be resistant to a given drug, the use of several different drugs tends to maximize effective cancer cell kill and minimize the kill of normal cells.

Chemotherapy is the treatment of choice for cancers that have spread or those that are normally disseminated throughout the body such as leukemias. While surgery and localized radiation therapy can only destroy localized cancers effectively, chemotherapy agents, by virtue of its total systemic nature, is active against cancer cells throughout the body. It is also highly effective in combination with surgery and/or radiation therapy to destroy cancer cells that have escaped the localized treatment.

Chemotherapeutic agents are normally administered by mouth or by injection into muscles or blood vessels. For fairly localized tumors this method has the disadvantage that the entire body is subject to the drug. With some cancers special techniques can be used to localize the effect. One example is direct injection into the tumor. Of great effectiveness is tissue perfusion. With this technique the drug is placed into blood vessels that lead directly to the cancerous organ or limb. The circulation is often bypassed, so that the return flow of blood is not to the heart or lungs but directly back to the perfusion system. In this way, high concentrations of antitumor drugs can be administered to the cancerous area for extended periods of time without significant hazard to the patient.

Remembering that antitumor drugs are most effective against cycling cells, one should expect considerable side effects to result from damage to the numerous types of cells in the body that are normally growing. These cells are less susceptible to radiation damage than to chemical damage, because radiation is rarely applied to the entire body, yet, as we have said, the drugs usually pervade all of the body except brain tissue. The particular types of cells that suffer are the cells surrounding hair roots (damage to which causes hair loss), blood-forming tissues in the spleen and bone marrow (resulting in anemia and a reduced immune response), and epithelial cells in the entire alimentary tract from the mouth to the rectum (causing tenderness, vomiting, diarrhea, and so forth). However, sufficient differences in the rate of regeneration of normal tissue versus tumor tissue makes chemotherapy effective if given in stages: drug treatment, a rest period for several days or weeks, drug treatment, etc.

We mentioned above that a single drug is usually not effective, especially for disseminated tumors. The effect of combining drugs in sequence can be seen best in the case of acute lymphocytic leukemia. Various single drugs, in repeated doses, were tried in the early years of chemotherapy, and a cure rate of no more than 1% was seen. However, a combination of four different drugs (affecting DNA synthesis in various ways, protein synthesis, and RNA synthesis) over a period of three years increases the cure rate to 25%. If during the period in which cancer cells seem to be absent (the remission induction phase) steroids and the mitotic inhibitor vincristine is given, remission is complete in about 90% of all patients. Again, if other drugs are then given, remission is maintained and 5-year survival rates of 100% have been achieved.

Combination chemotherapy (the use of more than one drug) is the most common type of chemotherapy. This type of treatment is effective for a variety of reasons, but mainly because the drugs used have different modes of action and provide a multifaceted attack on the cancer cells. Another reason is that cancer cells sometimes develop resistance to one of the chemicals, but seldom to more than one. In addition, one drug sometimes helps another drug to act. For example, vincristine helps cells take up methotrexate, so these two drugs are often given together.

Chemotherapeutic drugs are of a variety of types and they are classified according to their mode of action:

1. Antimetabolites are drugs that are structurally similar to compounds that are important to the life of a cell. These drugs, because of their resemblance to compounds that cells use, interfere with cellular processes by substituting for the useful compound. In this way, cellular reactions are inhibited because although the antimetabolite may enter a reaction, the reaction does not work effectively. An example of an antimetabolite is 5-fluorouracil, a compound resembling the DNA base thymine (a fluorine atom is present at the site of a methyl group in thymine). 5-Fluorouracil interferes with DNA synthesis and in quite a complex way causes death of cells attempting to synthesize DNA. 5-Fluorouracil is very effective in treating some forms of cancer of the digestive tract and breast. Another antimetabolite is methotrexate, which resembles the vitamin folic acid. Because of the role of folic acid in many biochemical reactions, methotrexate interferes with the synthesis of DNA, RNA, and protein. It is very effective in the treatment of certain uterine cancers, but is used mostly in combination with other drugs in treating leukemia, testicular cancer, and a large number of other organ tumors. It is an exceedingly valuable drug.

2. Alkylating agents, which developed from research on mustard gases during World War II, are drugs that react with various molecules essential to the life of cells, most commonly DNA. They cause severe errors in DNA replication, and thereby lead to the production of cells sufficiently defective that they cannot survive. Cyclophosphamide (cytoxan) is the most commonly used alkylating agent; it is quite

effective in the treatment of Hodgkin's disease, Burkitt's lymphoma, lymphosarcomas, neuroblastoma, and cancer of the breast, ovary, and lung. It has no affect on cells in culture, for it must be enzymatically converted in the liver to the active form.

3. Antimitotics are a group of compounds, usually isolated from plants of the species Vinca (hence, the common term vinca alkaloids), that interfere with formation of the mitotic spindle in cells. Chromosomes fail to separate into daughter cells in cells attempting to divide in the presence of these drugs, with the result that both daughter cells die. The most commonly used antimitotics are vinblastine and vincristine. These drugs are effective in treating gestational trophoblastic tumors, acute lymphoblastic leukemia, Hodgkin's disease, and breast carcinoma, and as a follow-up treatment in leukemia and after radiotherapy.

4. Antibiotics are compounds, usually synthesized by fungi and active against many bacteria, that are also effective against some cancer cells. Actinomycin D, an RNA synthesis inhibitor, is effective in treating Wilms' tumor in children and certain uterine cancer. Daunomycin, bleomycin, and adriamycin are two other effective anticancer antibiotics that appear to act by binding to DNA and preventing RNA synthesis. Adriamycin is very effective in treating leukemias, lymphomas, and other cancers.

5. Asparaginase is an enzyme that converts the amino acid asparagine to another amino acid, aspartic acid. Asparagine is not required by normal cells, because they can synthesize their own, but certain leukemia cells cannot make this amino acid. These cells need an external source of asparagine, such as the blood. Administration of large amounts of asparaginase to individuals with some types of childhood leukemia has been somewhat effective in treatment of the disease, presumably by eliminating the free asparagine in the blood and other body fluids. However, sometimes the leukemia cells become adapted to the lack of asparagine and begin to synthesize their own. Thus, the drug, when used alone, causes an apparent remission, but the disease returns.

Chemotherapy is most effective on continuously and rapidly dividing cancer cells, as we have said. It is far less effective against the many slow-growing cancers. However, a significant research effort is directed toward finding agents that can kill such slow growing cells effectively. This is a difficult problem because in such a tumor most of the cancer cells are not multiplying and hence are no more sensitive to antitumor agents than normal cells.

The growth of some tumors depends on the availability of certain hormones and tends to slow down if the level of these hormones in the body is reduced, or if the hormone is antagonized. For example, some ovarian tumors can be treated with male sex hormones or various antiestrogens. The steroid hormone, prednisone, is also useful in treating certain types of leukemia. However, hormonal approaches to treatment of some cancers have yielded variable results, because in time the tumor cells often lose their dependence on hormones.

The toxic side effects of chemotherapy have given it a bad name in the minds of many uninformed individuals. However, the statistics speak for themselves. That is, with proper use of chemotherapeutic agents many cures are achieved in patients who, not too long ago, would have been considered incurable.

Chemotherapeutic agents are continually under development and testing. Some of the agents are prepared as chemical variants of known agents; others are just randomly produced chemicals. The screening techniques in use by the government and by industry use a variety of systems, mainly transplantable leukemias, lung cancers, and skin tumors of mice. These tumors are injected into susceptible mice and then challenged with potential antitumor drugs. About 1 in every 1000 agents tested improves the life span of the mice by 25% or more, compared to mice that have not received the drug. Each potential drug is then extensively tested for toxicity in animals and finally in clinical trials with humans. Many years of testing usually are required before a drug can be used, and any drug that finally reaches the public is backed up by extensive testing for toxicity and effectiveness. The long-term survival of acute leukemia patients from 0 to more than 50 percent since the introduction of chemotherapeutic agents attests to the value of these agents.

COMBINED SURGERY, RADIATION, AND CHEMOTHERAPY

Combining surgery, radiation, and chemotherapy is often more successful than using one treatment alone. Some examples are preoperative irradiation to destroy peripheral tumor extensions, post-operative chemotherapy to destroy circulating cancer cells and cell clusters, post-irradiation surgery to remove residual tumor cells not destroyed by radiation, and a combination of surgery with other treatments such as chemotherapy, and/or radiotherapy, and/or stimulation of the immune system. The use of such combined treatments arose from the recognition that there are many types of cancer in which complete surgical excision of the primary tumor is possible, yet statistically the prognosis is poor. An example is breast cancer with lymph node metastases, in which the 5-year survival is only 10% even when all lymph nodes, both cancerous and noncancerous, are removed. The problem is that microscopic clusters of cells remain in the tumor area and that metastatic sites often have already been established elsewhere in the body. This is especially acute with very slow-growing tumors, since new growth may not appear until a considerable time has elapsed. However, for many of these breast cancers if radiation and chemotherapy are used after surgery at several intervals over the next year, the 5-year survival rate can be increased to >90%. Another striking example is Wilms' tumor, a kidney cancer of children, which has a cure rate of 23% from surgery alone, 40% when both surgery and radiotherapy are used, and more than 80% if following surgery and radiotherapy, actinomycin D is given. Osteogenic sarcoma is a bone cancer, also in children, with a very poor prognosis. In one study, half of the patients had metastatic tumors 5-9 months after surgery, but with high doses of methotrexate and another agent, 11 of 12 patients were free of tumors after a year. In another study of the same disease 14 of 15 patients remained free of the disease for two years when treated with adriamycin following surgery. As a result of these and other successes combinations of therapeutic procedures are being used with increasing frequency. At present, they have become routine for cancer of the oral cavity, embryonal rhabdo-myosarcoma, testicular cancer, and retinoblastoma.

IMMUNOTHERAPY

Immunotherapy means a variety of things: (1) administration of generalized immunostimulants, such as BCG (see Chapter 9), (2) production of cancer vaccines with living cancer cells or cancer antigens, (3) inoculating cancer patients with white blood cells that have been sensitized to specific cancer cells, (4) the use of interferon to activate killer cells, and (5) attempts to isolate informational molecules that may direct white blood cells to mount an immune response against specific cancers. So far, only item (1) has been used to any great extent. The other treatments, which will be mentioned in this section, are in developmental stages but appear promising. Furthermore, it seems unlikely at present that immunotherapy will, by itself, be used in treatment; more probably, it will be used in conjunction with other treatments.

BCG vaccine may be effective in treating some cancers. It is administered as a suspension of an attenuated strain of a tuberculosis bacterium and causes a general stimulation of the immune system. With certain animal tumors BCG has been effective in causing complete regression of tumors, for example, those produced by injecting tumor cells into guinea pigs. In one study, when BCG was not given, guinea pigs died with lymph node metastases 66 days after injection with tumor cells. With BCG added after the tumor began to form, the tumors regressed, and the animals were still alive a year after tumor cell injection, with no indication of tumor spread. In humans, direct injection of BCG into melanomas has been highly effective, as shown in Figure 13-6. When BCG is injected in combination with killed cancer cells, the reduction in the size of the tumor is even more striking. It is as if the killed cancer cells are triggering an immune response against surface antigens and the BCG activates the immune system, making the response very strong. BCG also appears to prolong disease-free periods in childhood leukemia patients who have been treated by chemotherapy. Similar results have been reported in patients with adult leukemia, Hodgkin's disease, skin cancer, certain colon cancers, and cancer of the head and neck. Injection of cell walls of Corynebacterium parvum (a bacterium related to the one that causes diphtheria), also a generalized immunostimulant, has helped shrink liver and lung cancers. In general, these stimulants are more effective in the treatment of small early human cancers than larger, more advanced tumors. However, they do show some promise in eliminating spread of tumors, if administered after the primary tumor has been removed surgically. The explanation given is that if a large tumor is present, the immune system will concentrate on cells of that tumor, so other cells in the body will be able to survive. If the primary tumor is removed, the defenses will be directed mostly against the other, more dangerous cells.

Another example of immunotherapy, which is being actively tested,

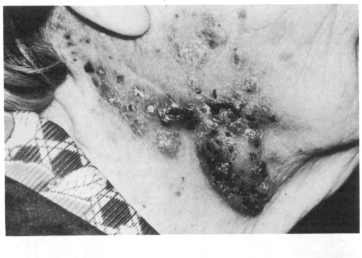

(a)

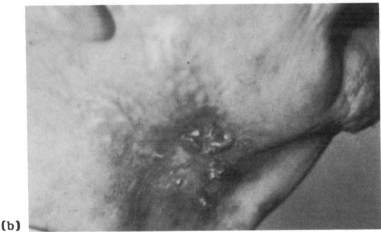

(b)

FIGURE 13-6 Use of immunotherapy in treatment of malignant melanoma. (a) before treatment. (b) One month later.

uses tumor cells taken from the patient. These cells are irradiated to kill them, and then treated with the enzyme neuraminidase, which removes a particular surface molecule (sialic acid) from the surfaces of the cells. The idea is that treatment of the cells with this enzyme will unmask tumor antigens from these cells (Figure 9-3). These treated cells are then injected back into the patient in the hopes of obtaining a strong immune response. Techniques such as this one coupled with injection with BCG have been somewhat effective against some cancers.

Combination of immunotherapy and chemotherapy is more effective than individual treatment. For example, in one study leukemia patients

received either chemotherapy alone or chemotherapy plus immunotherapy, and the patients in the latter group were free of the disease
for 50% longer than the patients receiving only chemotherapy. In this
study, immunotherapy consisted of inoculating patients with leukemia
cells treated with neuraminidase, as described in the preceding
paragraph.

A variety of new techniques are being studied and tested in a
limited way. One of these uses what has been called immune RNA,
an RNA species isolated from lymphoid tissues. Immune RNA has been
isolated from lymphocytes of humans who have been cured of melanoma;
this RNA appears able to stimulate other lymphocytes to attack
melanoma cells. Interestingly, the immune RNA can be extracted from
animals immunized with human melanoma cells, and the animal RNA can
stimulate human lymphocytes to kill human melanoma cells in culture.
It remains to be seen whether immune RNA will be of major clinical
importance. Another treatment uses a substances called thymosin, an
extract from the thymus gland of the cow. Thymosin stimulates T
cells to respond to antigens. It has shown promise in one type of
lung cancer, especially when used in combination with chemotherapy
and radiation therapy. Dinitrochlorobenzene is a fairly simple chemical
that causes a strong immune response. It has been painted on some
skin cancers and has been quite effective in eliminating the tumor.

In Chapter 9 we pointed that the body possesses various types
of cells that are able to kill tumor cells. Two new techniques, both
of which are in the experimental stage, are based on the activation
of these cells. These are administration of lymphokines and interferon.

Lymphokines are substances released by antigenically activated
lymphocytes. One of these, macrophage activation factor (MAF)
activates macrophages, cells that are able to destroy and engulf tumor
cells. In the past, the use of lymphokines has been limited by lack
of availability, since they are made in exceedingly small amounts.
However, new techniques of genetic engineering have made it possible
to synthesize large quantities in the laboratory, and they are now
being prepared by commercial bioengineering companies. The principal
difficulty with lymphokines is how to administer them. If they are
injected into the body, they quickly get diluted by body fluids to
such an extent that enormous amounts would have to be given in
order to activate the macrophages. However, an ingenious technique
allows them to be delivered directly to the target cells, the
macrophages themselves. A familiar observation is the formation of
small droplets of oil when oil and water are shaken together. A similar
effect can be seen with natural fats and their component molecules,
lipids. By use of appropriate conditions small lipid droplets can be
prepared which are hollow. These hollow droplets are called liposomes.
If liposomes are formed in solutions of lymphokines, the resulting
liposomes are filled with the lymphokines. Liposomes are quite stable
and can be injected directly into the bloodstream of an animal. Recall
that macrophages have the ability to engulf cells and small particles.
When a macrophage encounters a circulating liposome, it engulfs it.
Enzymes in the macrophage break down the lipid wall, and the contents
of the liposome are released into the cytoplasm of the macrophage.
Hence, if liposomes are injected that contain MAF, macrophages will

receive the major part of the administered MAF and become active killers of tumor cell. This technique has been tested in mice inoculated with malignant melanoma cells. Without other treatment 90% of the mice developed metastases. However, if liposomes containing MAF were given three days after injection with the melanoma cells and the treatment was continued twice a week for three weeks, only 27% developed metastases, indicating the potential value of this treatment in humans. More animal tests and some human tests are now in progress.

Interferons, as described briefly in Chapter 9, are a class of proteins synthesized in response to infection with most viruses and which have antiviral activity. There are several types of interferons made by different cells. The interferon formed by activated T cells, called immune interferon, is a modulator of the immune system and shows some antitumor activity. Although the activity of interferons was recognized some years ago, detailed experiments were impossible because of the tiny quantities available. However, with the recent cloning of several interferon genes by genetic engineering techniques 100% pure interferon is now being commercially produced and tested widely. Its mode of action against cancer cells is not known, but it is clear that it functions by activating the natural killers (NK) cells. Whether it makes old NK cells more active toward tumor cells or causes synthesis of new NK cells is not known. However, at present the reasons are unimportant: enough examples of clinical remission of cancers have been observed to warrant continued testing. So far, remissions have been observed with myeloma, non-Hodgkin's lymphoma, osteogenic sarcoma, and malignant melanoma, and a definite lengthening of life in advanced breast cancer. When interferon was first tested, it was thought to be a "magic bullet" that would defeat cancer. The actual clinical picture has been less encouraging: it has not proved to be effective against all cancers, and there have been a variety of undesirable side effects. On the positive side, the side effects were observed mostly with impure samples (less than 1% pure), and it is hoped that with the highly purified samples available today by genetic engineering, many of the side effects might disappear.

Interferon also directly inhibits the growth of many tumor cells in culture. In contrast with most chemotherapeutic agents, which act on dividing cells, it seems to act primarily on nondividing tumor cells, with only minimal effect on nondividing normal cells. Possibly, when used in conjunction with a chemotherapeutic agent, interferon will provide the ability to kill the resting cells in a tumor, which are normally unaffected in chemotherapy. Recall that chemotherapy must normally be given over a prolonged period of time (with all the attendant side effects) in order to allow time for nondividing tumor cells to enter the division phase. Possibly, a single dose, or a small number of doses, or a mixture of interferon and a drug will be more effective than the drug alone and will significantly decrease the time required for treatment.

Cancer cells, like all cells, possess transplantation antigens on their surfaces. These antigens result in rejection of cells when cells are injected into another individual: for example, a heart transplant is rejected by a recipient with a tissue type different from that of the donor, unless drugs are given to suppress the immune response.

These antigens can be made use of in immunotherapy of cancer. For example, cancer cells from patient X could be used to produce an anticancer vaccine for patient Y, but patient Y will reject the cancer cells from patient X. However, during the rejection reaction patient Y will also produce antibody and T cell populations that can react with the <u>tumor-associated antigens</u> on the cancer cells (Figure 13-7). Other white blood cell populations will react to the tissue transplantation antigens on the cells from patient X. In this way, patient Y will reject the cancer cells of patient X, so that these cells will not produce a cancer in patient Y. However, patient Y will also build up an immunity against the tumor-associated antigens. In this way, injection of cancer cells from X might result in regression of a tumor in Y or prevent future tumors from developing. This technique is currently being tested.

Another novel immunological technique, in the earliest stages of testing, is the use of <u>monoclonal antibodies,</u> which are pure samples

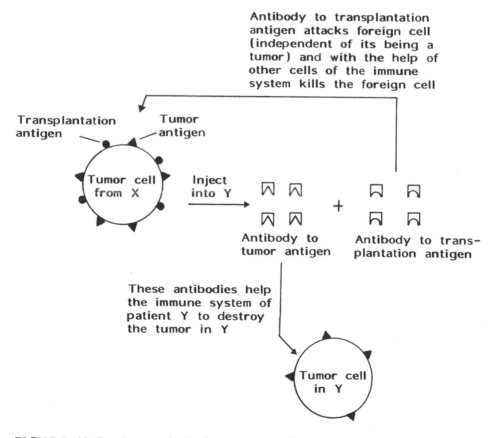

FIGURE 13-7   Immunological response of a recipient (patient Y) to injection of a tumor cell from another person (X).

of an antibody directed against a single antigen. Monoclonal antibodies are derived from clones of a single antibody-producing cell, whereas typical antibody isolates are derived from many different cells and are a mixture of tens of thousands of different antibodies. Therefore, monoclonals (a common abbreviation) are completely homogeneous and have extraordinary sensitivity in targeting their respective antigens. Monoclonals are obtained by fusing normal lymphocytes (antibody-producing cells) with a myeloma cancer cell line (an immortalized cell), yielding hybrid cells called hybridomas. Each hybridoma cell line grows indefinitely and produces a single specific antibody. By probing with a particular antigen it is possible to find a hybridoma that makes a desired antibody. Hybridoma technology permits the production of abundant pure antibodies that have a variety of uses. Pertinent to cancer is the ability to detect specific tumor antigens. Monoclonal antibodies are currently being used in cancer diagnosis and treatment. Many bioengineering companies are devoted solely to the production of monoclonal antibodies, and a variety of monoclonals are available.

Of particular interest are the monoclonals directed against particular tumor antigens, and several approaches are being taken to use these monoclonals in cancer treatment. A direct treatment would be to administer a monoclonal antibody against a tumor antigen in the hopes of destroying tumor cells directly. This does not work, though in experimental animals tumor cells circulating in the blood and lymph are eliminated. Other approaches use the ability of a monoclonal to target a tumor cell and carry a toxic substance directly to the cell. For example, monoclonal antibodies to carcinoembryonic antigen, which is made by certain liver cancers, has been made highly radioactive by coupling with iodine-131 in the laboratory. Injection of this radioactive monoclonal presumably delivers the radioactive atom to the surface of the liver cancer cells; because of the specificity of the antibody, no other cells should be affected. Indeed, the use of this radioactive monoclonal has produced clinical remissions in some liver cancer patients. A related technique uses a monoclonal antibody directed against a tumor antigen derived from Lewis lung carcinoma in the mouse. The antibody was coupled to a potent antitumor drug, daunorubicin, which by itself has limited effective against cancer (though it is useful in combined chemotherapy). In a preliminary test the monoclonal-daunorubicin complex was injected into mice with Lewis lung carcinoma, and a significant reduction in death and metastasis plus an increase in the lifetime of the animals were observed. Bacterial toxins, such as diphtheria toxin, and plant toxins, such as ricin (all of which are powerful inhibitors of protein synthesis in mammalian cells), have also been coupled to monoclonals and have shown some effectiveness against animal cancers. In another study monoclonals were produced against the surface antigens of mouse melanoma B16 cells. These antibodies blocked adhesion of these cells to culture vessels and also greatly inhibited colonization of these cells to the lung when the cells were injected into an animal. That is, the monoclonals blocked lung metastases by B16 melanoma cells. Monoclonals against hepatitis B virus surface antigens, present in a line of human hepatoma cells, specifically destroyed human hepatoma cells and suppressed tumor formation when the cells were injected into mice.

A monoclonal known as Fib-75 binds to an antigen present on cells from all tumors of organ surfaces (epithelial tumors) and kills these cells without harming normal cells. This antibody is being used in a dramatic way. When cancer patients are given massive doses of whole-body radiation and chemotherapy to kill cancer cells, they often lose all of their bone marrow cells, which virtually eliminates their immune system. However, samples of marrow can be removed prior to treatment and then returned to the bone to recolonize the marrow (see next section). Unfortunately, the marrow often contains cancer cells that have spread from the primary tumor. Treatment of the isolated marrow with Fib-75 frees the marrow of cancer cells. Thus, when the marrow is returned to the patient, the immune system of these patients can be regenerated without reestablishing the cancer. These new techniques are obviously being studied intensively in many laboratories and clinics.

BONE MARROW TRANSPLANTS

Bone marrow transplantation is a special surgical treatment used in certain cases of leukemia, aplastic anemia and other bone marrow cancers. In treating these diseases it is necessary to destroy the patient's entire bone marrow to eliminate the cancer cells. This is done with high doses of drugs and radiation. Without any marrow the patient would be unable to manufacture antibodies and would die of bacterial or viral infection (or else be forced to live in a sterile environment). However, the fatality can in theory be eliminated by a marrow transplant. Only certain individuals are candidates for transplants because of the problem of rejection of foreign tissue. The patient must have siblings or other possible donors who possess similar tissue antigen types. If the new bone marrow is different with respect to certain surface antigens (transplantation antigens), the immune cells produced by the donor's marrow will consider most of the tissues of the recipient (the patient) to be foreign and will destroy the tissue. Thus, unlike kidney and heart transplants, which may be rejected by the immune system of the recipient, with a poorly matched bone marrow transplant, the transplant (which produces immune cells) will reject the recipient; this is called graft versus host disease.

Assuming that a suitable donor is available, bone marrow transplantation is still usually used only when other therapies prove unsuccessful. Donor marrow is removed with a syringe and transfused into the bloodstream of the recipient (after the recipient's own marrow has been destroyed). The marrow cells find their way to the bones and colonize them. All of the precursor cells that form red and white blood cells are present in the marrow of the donor, so the recipient becomes able to produce all cell types needed for survival. Three complications may occur. (1) All of the cancer cells might not be destroyed. (2) The recipient may die of infection before the new marrow is functional. To reduce the latter problem, patients are kept in sterile chambers and are transfused with whole blood until their own marrow is adequate. (3) The graft-induced host rejection is always a problem, but drugs are available that reduce the effect. In certain cases, for example, when monoclonal antibodies are used to destroy host cancer cells, as described in the preceding section, a small portion of the patient's own marrow can be used to recolonize the marrow, thus avoiding graft versus host disease.

Bone marrow transplantation offers promise in the treatment of some solid cancers such as breast cancer. Often the cancer is so widespread that massive doses of chemotherapeutic drugs are needed, and these drugs destroy the marrow cells. An approach that is being tried to avoid this problem is to remove the patient's marrow (which may not contain cancer cells) before drug treatment and freeze it in liquid nitrogen. Once the drug therapy program is completed, the marrow is restored to the patient. This treatment is in the experimental stage.

ANTIANGIOGENESIS FACTORS

Recall that an important stage of development of a cancer is the ingrowth of blood vessels into the newly formed tumor. Without such vascularization, limitation of availability of nutrients prevents the tumor from growing to more than a few millimeters in diameter. If capillary ingrowth could be prevented. the development of both primary and secondary tumors would be severely restricted. Inhibitors of vascularization have been isolated from cartilage and the vitreous humor of the eye, but because of their limited availability, these inhibitors have not yet been well characterized. Recently, protamine, a commercially available substance isolated from sperm of all animals, has been found to inhibit capillary growth in embryos, in certain inflammation and immune reactions, and in solid tumors.

In the early studies of angiogenesis it was observed that a combination of heparin (an anticoagulant) and an angiogenesis promoter isolated from tumor tissue caused extensive vascularization, far greater than with the promoter alone. When protamine, which binds to heparin is added, growth of capillaries into tumors is prevented. In an important experiment, mice were injected with lung cancer cells and a sufficient time was allowed to form a primary tumor. Protamine was then injected. This treatment resulted in a 97% inhibition of lung metastases, and it seems likely that the antitumor activity of protamine resulted from its ability to bind heparin. Unfortunately protamine is fairly toxic to animals, though not to cells growing in culture. In another experiment heparin plus the hormone cortisone was found to cause large tumors in mice to shrink, and metastasis was prevented. The combination of these drugs appeared to work by preventing capillary growth to the expanding tumor. The responsive tumors were reticulum cell carcinomas, Lewis lung carcinomas, and B16 melanomas. The combined data from several tumors showed 4553 lung metastases in 73 untreated animals versus only 3 metastases in 39 treated animals. The antitumor effects of heparin plus cortisone were better than any known inhibitor of capillary growth. It remains to be seen whether this therapy will be as effective in humans as in mice.

Protamine has been used experimentally in England for treating breast cancers in humans and animals with a modicum of success. Although control of tumor angiogenesis has not reached the point of major clinical utility, these studies suggest that it may be a valuable procedure.

LAETRILE

Since laetrile has been the subject of a great deal of interest in recent years, it is appropriate to mention some of the factual information that deals with the use of this substance in cancer treatment.

Laetrile is made from apricot pits and is a registered trade mark for the compound amygdalin present in the seeds of many plants. It was originally proposed that laetrile could kill cancer cells by release of cyanide in the cells. Supporters of laetrile treatment believe that cancer cells contain large amounts of an enzyme that releases cyanide from amygdalin and that normal cells contain much smaller amounts of this enzyme. There is little reason at this point to discuss the proposed biochemical effects of laetrile and the reasons that it was considered by its proponents to be the most effective treatment for cancer, because there is now no doubt that it is completely ineffective. Numerous series of carefully controlled experiments in animals were sponsored by the U.S. National Cancer Institute over a period of 30 years and more recently to test the effects of laetrile on a variety of animal tumors. In all of the experiments, when the results were evaluated by objective criteria, laetrile failed to reduce the growth of cancers. No unbiased, objective, reproducible work suggests that laetrile is effective against animal tumors.

Clinical tests of laetrile have been carried out with thousands of humans at major cancer centers in the United States. Many of the patients were also given special "health-food" diets including large doses of vitamins and minerals, as recommended by proponents of laetrile. In no case, has laetrile, or laetrile plus a special diet, been shown to be of any value in either curing or extending life. Isolated examples of cures advertised by the proponents of laetrile are statistically insignificant and represent the recovery rate expected following previous treatment or without any treatment at all. There is no doubt that laetrile should not be used in the treatment of any cancer. After completing an extensive series of tests, Dr. Vincent DeVita, head of the U.S. National Cancer Institute, stated, "The hollow promise of this drug has led thousands of Americans away from potentially helpful therapy of scientific validity. Now the facts speak for themselves."

SUMMARY

Many localized cancers are curable with surgery or radiation therapy. A variety of disseminated cancers are curable with chemotherapy. However, many metastasized cancers cannot be effectively treated, and cures are achieved only in a rather modest percentage of cases. Thus, the major problem in cancer treatment is in metastatic cancer. However, encouraging results with combined radiation and chemotherapy and with immunotherapy are beginning to emerge, and there is reason for optimism that many widespread cancers, presently resistant to treatment, may eventually be curable. Improved diagnostic methods, too, will in all probability lead to earlier cancer diagnosis before spread has occurred. If this proves correct, conventional forms of treatment will cure many more cancers than they do today, because the tumors will have been identified before spread has occurred. Numerous novel techniques, still in the experimental stage, seem quite promising.

ADDITIONAL READINGS

Bochow, A. 1976. "Cancer immunotherapy: What promise does it hold?" Nursing, 76, 50.

Burchenal, J.H., and J.R. Burchenal. 1977. "Chemotherapy of cancer." Chemistry 50.

Frei III, E. 1982. "The National Cancer Chemotherapy Program." Science, 217, 600.

Marshall, E. 1982. "Gambling on interferon." Science, 216, 1078.

Morra, M., and Potts, E. 1980. Choices.: Realistic Alternatives in Cancer Treatment. Avon.

Moss, W. T., W.N. Brand, and H. Bothford. 1973. Radiation Oncology: Rationale, Technique, Results. C. V. Mosby.

Nelson, D. F., and P. Rubin. 1977. "Radiation therapy." Chemistry 50.

Patterson, B. 1974. Principles of Surgical Oncology. Clinical Oncology for Medical Students and Physicians.

Pinkel, D. 1971. "Five-year follow-up of "total therapy" of childhood lymphocytic leukemia." J. Am. Med. Assoc. 216, 648.

Prosuitz, L. R. 1971. "Radiation therapy." RN Magazine.

Rhoads, C. P. 1948. "Weeds and grass--an analogy". Sloan-Kettering Institute Annual Report.

Rubin, P. 1974. Principles of Radiation Therapy. Clinical Oncology for Medical Students and Physicians.

Ruddon, R.W. 1981. Cancer Biology. Chapter 8. Oxford.

Schafer, L.A., and E.M. Hersh. 1977. "Immunotherapy of human cancer." Chemistry 50.

Shouvall, D., D.A. Shafritz, V.R. Zurawski, K.J. Isselbacher, and J.R. Wands. 1982. "Immunotherapy in nude mice of human hepatoma using monoclonal antibodies against hepatitis B virus." <u>Nature</u>, 298, 567.

Thorpe, P.E., D.W. Mason, A.N.F. Brown, S.J. Simmonds, W.C.J. Ross, A.J. Cumber, and J.A. Forrester. 982. "Selective killing of malignant cells in a leukemic rat bone marrow using an antibody-rich conjugate." <u>Nature,</u> 297, 594.

Vollmers, H.P. and W. Birchmeier. 1983. "Monoclonal antibodies inhibit the adhesion of mouse B16 melanoma cells in vitro and block lung metastasis in vivo." <u>Proc. Nat. Acad. Sci.</u>, 80, 3729.

<u>Treating Cancer</u>. 1972. HEW Monograph.

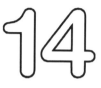

Protection
Against Cancer

So far, we have been concerned primarily with the cellular and clinical manifestations of cancer. In this chapter we will look at how individuals may be able to protect themselves from getting cancer.

Throughout this text we have seen examples of numerous cancer-causing agents. Now we will bring this and other information together to develop a reasonable personal program that may be valuable in preventing some forms of cancer in some individuals. It has been estimated that of the approximately 400,000 people in the United States who die of cancer each year, 200,000 or more of these deaths are avoidable using currently understood strategies for cancer prevention. There is little doubt that the subject of cancer prevention will become of major importance in reducing cancer deaths in the near future. A summary of the actions that can be taken that may reduce the risk of developing cancer will be presented in this chapter; however, one must be careful to recognize that many of these actions are inferred from animal tests, laboratory experiments, and statistical analyses of human populations and have yet to be proved to be a means of prevention of human cancer. Possibly it will take a long time to demonstrate with certainty that some of these strategies are indeed effective; however, in the meantime it is prudent to take the actions.

Cancer prevention is not a new subject. That some cancers could be prevented was first recognized in England in the 18th century when Percival Pott noticed that patients with scrotal cancer had all been chimney sweeps as children. These children crawled through chimneys with no clothes, and coal soot, now known to contain numerous carcinogens, would lodge in the folds of the scrotum. Pott introduced the practice of wearing clothes and frequent bathing, and the incidence of this type of cancer became very low.

SENSIBLE STRATEGIES FOR MINIMIZING THE RISK OF CANCER

There are two aspects to reducing the risk of death by cancer: (1) preventing cancer and (2) early detection to avoid advanced cancer. In this section we begin by describing a variety of accepted strategies for cancer prevention.

Smoking

Smoking is the most important single cause of cancer in the U.S. More than 100,000 people die of lung cancer each year (25% of all cancer deaths), and most of these deaths result from cigarette smoking. In addition, the incidence of cancer of the bladder, larynx, oral cavity, esophagus, kidney, and other parts of the body is significantly increased by regular smoking. Why this is the case is illustrated in Table 14-1, which lists agents found in cigarette smoke that are known from laboratory and animal tests to be carcinogens. Most of these substances are synthesized by the tobacco plant itself. A few, the metals and metallic compounds, are picked up from the soil and concentrated in the leaves. These substances exert their effect by virtue of their chemical properties. Even a radioactive element, polonium-210, is present; it is concentrated in the tobacco leaf by tiny hairs that pick up small amounts of this element naturally

TABLE 14-1   Known carcinogens found in tobacco or in cigarette smoke

Aminostilbene	N-Dibutylnitrosoamine
Arsenic	2,3-Dimethylchrysene
Benz-(a)-anthracene	Indenol-(1,2,3-cd)-pyrene
Benz-(a)-pyrene	5-Methylchrysene
Benzene	Methylfluoranthrene
Benzo-(b)-fluoranthrene	β-Naphthylamine
Benzo-(c)-phenanthrene	Nickel compounds
Cadmium	N-Nitrosomethylethylamine
Chrysene	N-Nitrosodiethylamine
Dibenz-(a,h)-acridie	N-Nitrosonanabasine
Dibenz-(a,j)-acridine	N-Nitrosopiperidine
Dibenz-(a,c)-anthracene	N-Nitrosopyrrolidine
Dibenz-(c,g)-carbazone	Polonium-210
Dibenz-(a,e)-fluoranthrene	

present in the soil. It is important to recognize that these substances are found not only in smoke, but also in chewing tobacco and snuff, which accounts for the extraordinary incidence of cancer of the mouth among users of chewing tobacco.

Note that by the simple (but really not so simple) expediency of eliminating all use of tobacco, more than 25,000 lives would not be lost every year, and this number does not include those dying of heart attacks and kidney disease, both of which occur at a significantly higher frequency among smokers.

Consumption of Alcohol

Excessive drinking of alcoholic beverages contributes to a variety of human disorders, among them, cancer. The incidence of cancer of the mouth, throat, larynx, esophagus, liver, and possibly the rectum is associated with heavy consumption of alcoholic beverages. Among smokers who also drink to excess, cancers of the esophagus and mouth are especially prevalent. Moderation (not necessary elimination) in the use of alcoholic beverage should decrease the risk of these cancers.

Dietary Considerations

That the risk of cancer correlates with diet has been known for many years. Two important studies involved the Japanese. When the Japanese migrated to the United States, abandoning their traditional diet, their rates of certain cancers, such as that of the colon-rectum region, breast, and prostate, increased, and others (described in Table 11-3) decreased. The cancers that increased seem to be associated with high consumption of fats, which constitute a major part of the diet in the U.S. and a minor part in Japan. Those that decreased are associated with eating smoked, salted, and pickled foods.

When considering the effect of diet on cancer, one must distinguish between those carcinogens that are naturally present in foods and those that are either added or arise as a result of processing or storage of foods. Furthermore, one must examine the ingestion of potential anticarcinogens and of substances that accelerate the elimination of ingested carcinogens. For example, it has been argued that we consume about 10,000 times more natural plant toxins (some of which are carcinogens) than manmade chemical contaminants. Plants have evolved a variety of poisons that defend against bacterial attack, mold growth, and invasion by other microorganisms. Some of these toxins that may be weakly carcinogenic or may enhance carcinogen activity include: safrole and piperine (in black pepper), hydrazines (in mushrooms), psoralen derivatives (in celery, figs, parsley, and parsnips), allyl isothiocyanate (in horseradish and oil of mustard), and theobromine (in chocolate and tea). There is no proof at present that ingestion of these foods can enhance the risk of cancer, but cutting down on foods containing these agents might be prudent.

The National Research Council, in its document, "Report on Diet, Nutrition, and Cancer," suggested that high fat consumption may be the most important dietary factor associated with increased cancer risk. Fat breakdown products and conditions in the intestine resulting from fat digestion may contribute to cancer risk. The body needs small amounts of fats, so it is unwise to attempt to eliminate all fat from the diet. However, reducing consumption by switching from fatty to lean meats and from high-fat dairy products to low-fat products is advisable. This will also have the beneficial effect of reducing the incidence of heart disease and stroke.

Most salt-cured and salt-pickled foods, such as salami, bologna, bacon, ham, and hot dogs, contain the preservative sodium nitrite. This substance is added to prevent the growth of bacteria and molds, many of which are harmful (and may even produce carcinogens). However, in the body or under conditions of high heat (such as frying bacon), nitrite combines with products of protein breakdown, called amines, to form nitrosamines, which are carcinogenic (Chapter 6). Therefore, it is wise to reduce the consumption of such foods, which are also high in fat content. It has been found that vitamin C is able to block the formation of nitrosamine from nitrite. Thus, since many people will find it nearly impossible to eliminate cured meats from their diet, it seems reasonable to couple ingestion of foods containing nitrites with consumption of foods rich in vitamin C, such as citrus fruits.

Several molds produce powerful carcinogens, such as aflatoxin and sterigmatocystin. Those found on the classical moldy cheeses are safe, but the molds that appear on peanut skins (black spots) and on whole grains stored in damp areas may be exceedingly dangerous. In general, except for the cheeses, moldy foods should be strictly avoided. U.S. government agencies carefully screen all grains, peanuts, soybeans, and peanut butter for aflatoxin. At one time, it was thought that the high incidence of stomach cancer in Japan was a result of aflatoxin produced by molds present on the stored soybeans used in the manufacture of soy sauce. This suspicion made people wary of the use of soy sauce and other soy products. A recent study in Japan has indicated that neither soy sauce nor any other soy food is the offending substance, which still remains to be discovered. It is currently thought to be some substance(s) in smoked, pickled, or salted food.

We pointed out earlier that cigarette smoke contains a large number of carcinogens present in tobacco. Other carcinogens are produced from harmless substances in tobacco by the act of burning. These same substances are present in the browned coatings of smoked, charred, heavily browned, and burned foods. Many authorities would consider it wise to change cooking styles of such foods.

In an earlier chapter in which tests for carcinogens were described, it was pointed out that many substances are not themselves carcinogenic, but are converted to carcinogens in the liver. Although there is a certain amount of debate, there seems to be enough reliable evidence to suggest that consumption of antioxidants may reduce these conversions and thereby decrease the risk of cancer. As a result of these studies increased consumption of fruits and vegetables rich in beta-carotene (a vitamin A precursor), vitamin A, and vitamin C has been recommended. Foods rich in these substances are acorn squash, apricots, broccoli, Brussel sprouts, cantaloupe, carrots, chard, collards, cress, dandelion leaves, endive, grapefruit, hubbard squash, kale, mustard greens, oranges, persimmon, pumpkin, and strawberries. Vitamin E, present in whole grain products, some meat, milk, and many vegetables, may also be effective. Consumption of tiny amounts of the mineral selenium, which may destroy carcinogenic peroxides, is also recommended; it is found in most balanced diets and is prevalent in bread, broccoli, Brussel sprouts, cabbage, cauliflower, fish, and rice.

Ingested carcinogens and substances made carcinogenic in the body often build up in the intestine and probably are a major cause of cancer of the intestine and colon. This problem can probably be reduced by an appropriate diet. Fruits, vegetables, and whole-grain products are generally high in indigestible materials collectively called fiber (once called bulk). Fiber maintains looseness of the intestinal contents, thereby speeding the passage of food wastes and leaving less time for buildup of carcinogens and their action of the intestinal wall. It also results in the formation of soft stools that are easily eliminated. The value of high-fiber diets is indicated by the very low incidence of colon-rectum cancer in countries in which the people have high-fiber diets consisting of grains, fruits, and vegetables. Thus, it is valuable to increase the amount of fiber-rich foods in the diet. Increasing the consumption of liquids (in particular, water) is also useful in diluting carcinogens and minimizing their transit time through the intestine.

A Comment about Vitamin A

Recently considerable attention has been given to the potential role of vitamin A in the prevention of certain cancers. Although definitive proof is not yet available, indirect evidence suggests that vitamin A and related substances (retinoids) might be valuable. Vitamin A plays a role in the maintenance of normal growth and development of tissues that line the surfaces of the body (epithelial tissues). In laboratory experiments in which vitamin A is eliminated, these tissues undergo processes of altered growth and differentiation similar to those that occur when the tissues are exposed to carcinogens. Vitamin A and its analogues can inhibit the development of chemically induced cancers in a variety of laboratory animals and and at several anatomical sites. Dietary deficiency of vitamin A in rats and mice also enhances their susceptibility to chemical carcinogens. Furthermore, some human social and ethnic groups, whose diets include only very small amounts of vitamin A, have a higher incidence of lung and bladder cancer.

Retinoids and vitamin A have also been used successfully in cancer therapy, particularly in the treatment of basal cell carcinomas of the skin and a variety of precancerous lesions.

A variety of detailed laboratory studies have indicated that vitamin A may prevent the induction of some cancers by one or more of the following mechanisms:

1. Direct binding of carcinogens.
2. Retinoid-induced cell-surface alterations (such as synthesis of sugar-containing molecules), which either interfere with the action of carcinogens at the cell surface or prevent expression of altered growth patterns.
3. Retinoid-caused inhibition of certain enzymes (for example, ornithine decarboxylase), which are required for cell proliferation.
4. Direct action of retinoids on the cell nucleus, leading to altered gene expression.
5. Retinoid-induced release of lysosomal enzymes, which may alter cellular interactions and may activate macrophages that possibly contribute to the destruction of developing cancer cells.

Although much more study is necessary, there is reason to think that vitamin A and its derivatives may be useful in both prevention and treatment of some human cancers.

Other Potential Agents for Preventing Cancer

A few agents other than vitamin A also show potential in cancer prevention. One example is alpha-aminocaproic acid, a specific inhibitor of the group of proteases called plasminogen activators (Chapter 4). When given to mice in drinking water, this substance reduces by a factor of 10 the incidence of colorectal tumors induced by injection of the carcinogen 1,2-dimethylhydrazine. Other important substances are BHT (butylated hydroxytoluene) and BHA (butylated hydroxyanisole), both used as food preservatives to maintain flavor, and the antiinflammatory drug indomethacin; these have been found to inhibit cancers produced by chemical carcinogens. How these agents work is not known. Prevention of cancer by use of various chemicals will in all likelihood offer new approaches to effective reduction of the incidence of cancer.

Exposure to Carcinogenic Chemicals at Home

Many chemicals found in the home are either known carcinogens or possible carcinogens, and exposure to them should be avoided. If work with them is necessary, the following measures will help to reduce exposure: protective clothing, frequent bathing, use of dust masks, use of respirators, and adequate ventilation.

Some paint pigments contain chemical compounds of nickel, chromium, cadmium, and arsenic, many of which are carcinogenic; one must never breathe in these substances when dissolving dry pigment. Cleaning solvents may contain benzene, carbon tetrachloride, trichloroethylene, and tetrachloroethylene, which are also weak carcinogens. Aerosols are especially hazardous, because they are easily inhaled in substantial quantities. Chemicals in some of the older permanent hair dyes test positively as mutagens in bacterial tests and may be carcinogenic when used over long periods or at high concentrations. Many modern hair dyes and other cosmetics contain substances that have not yet been tested adequately. In general, it is prudent to minimize the use of cosmetics and to examine product labels carefully. Never use products containing the dyes 2,4-toluenediamine and 4-methoxy-m-phenylenediamine, as these are known carcinogens.

A few drugs are also hazardous, as they are weak carcinogens. Nonetheless, they have been approved for public use when a good substitute is not available and the consequences of not using the drug are greater than the cancer risk. Table 14-2 lists several medicines that have in some tests shown weak carcinogenic activity; since substitutes are available, they should probably not be used. Taking estrogens or diethylstilbesterol (DES), an agent once used to prevent pregnancy, for menopausal discomfort should be avoided. If menopausal problems are severe or if other conditions require the use of estrogen therapy, it is best to try to use the smallest amount possible for the briefest time.

A variety of organic carcinogens and substances called "precarcinogens" are present in the drinking water of many U.S. cities. Among theses are benzene, chloromethyl ether, vinyl chloride, DDT, dieldrin, hexachlorocyclohexane, bis-(2-chloroethyl)-ether, carbon tetrachloride, heptachlor, pentachlorobiphenyl, carbon disulfide, and chloroform. The amounts are very small, and studies are underway that are designed to determine if the concentrations in municipal water supplies are related to increased risk of cancer. Both the Environmental Protection Agency and a leading consumer testing organization have shown that a variety of activated carbon filters,

TABLE 14-2   Substances used in medicine having carcinogenic activity in the laboratory

Substance	Use
Coal tar ointments	Skin disease
Flagyl	Vaginal infections
Griseofulvin	Scalp ringworm, athlete's foot
Lindane shampoos	Head lice
Phenacetin	Headache, pain killer

when used properly, can remove most of these substances from water. It cannot be said with certainty, but use of such filters may be helpful in reducing cancer risk, especially in those areas in which the contamination is especially high.

Exposure to Carcinogens at Work

Workers in a variety of occupations are exposed to chemical carcinogens of many types. Increased regulation of these industries (not yet done, in most cases) is necessary in order to reduce exposure. However, if workers become aware of the carcinogenicity of some of the chemicals with which they work, they may be able to reduce exposure themselves by using face masks and respirators, by changing work clothing at home, and by frequent bathing. Problem chemicals and industries are listed in Table 14-3.

Radiation Exposure

There is no doubt that the major cause of skin cancer is overexposure to ultraviolet radiation (UV) from sunlight. The incidence of skin cancer is higher in sunny regions of the United States (Florida, Arizona) and among people whose exposure to sunlight is especially high (compulsive tanners and outdoor workers). Fair-skinned individuals are particularly susceptible to the harmful effects of UV. All skin contains a protective pigment, called melanin, that absorbs UV and thereby prevents the deeper layers of the skin from being damaged. The skin of dark-skinned individuals contains more melanin than that of fair-skinned people. Tanning occurs when melanin-producing cells are stimulated to produce melanin granules that spread throughout the surface of the skin. Individuals who do not tan easily (or not at all) do not produce melanin in adequate quantities; thus, UV is not blocked, and burning occurs. UV can cause considerable damage to DNA; a variety of repair systems correct this damage, but some damage may persist and transform a normal cell to a cancer cell. Individuals with the disease xeroderma pigmentosum lack certain repair systems and have a high incidence of skin cancer.

Overexposure to sun is preventable by wearing protective clothing or using a variety of effective sunscreens (lotions, creams, etc.) The commonly used chemical in sunscreens are cinnamates, benzophenones, padimate O, salicylates, and p-aminobenzoic acid (PABA). The latter is considered by many skin specialists to be the most effective sunscreen, especially when present in an alcohol base and applied one hour before exposure to the sun. These substances absorb UV just like melanin does, block burning, and thereby prevent the DNA damage that may lead to cellular transformation. Most sunscreens contain only one of these substances; "tanning" lotions or oil that contain none of these substances are of no medicinal value. The public health department of the city of Honolulu officially reminds residents and tourists alike in local newspapers to use sunscreens at all times. Sunscreens in a base that forms a plastic film that does not come off in water are especially valuable.

X rays and the emission from radioactive materials also damage

DNA and are carcinogenic. Unnecessary exposure is prudent. However, the word unnecessary must be kept in mind, for x rays are critically important in diagnosing a variety of diseases and damaging conditions. Only the completely routine x ray should be questioned. When x rays are needed, it is advisable to ask about the age of the equipment used. Modern equipment delivers far lower radiation doses than older units and is widespread in hospitals and major medical services. In all cases, protective devices should be worn when possible in order to reduce the exposure to neighboring parts of the body.

Pregnant (and possibly pregnant) women should not be x-irradiated unless absolutely necessary, because embryonic tissues are especially susceptible to radiation damage. The risk of some types of cancer, and especially leukemia, is increased in children who were exposed to x rays in the womb.

In several cases, x rays are essential in early detection of cancer, for example, chest x rays for lung cancer and CAT scans for a variety of tumors. Mammography is especially valuable in detection of early breast cancer, even before tumors are detectible by physical examinations. Older equipment required a fairly high dose, but newer equipment delivers a dose that is sufficiently small that there is probably no significant risk. It is clearly important to ascertain that modern equipment delivering a dose between 1/25 and 1/3 rad is being used.

Environmental radiation from radioactive material has been of concern for some years, especially since the establishment of nuclear power plants. However, the level of radioactivity caused by human activity is, excluding diagnostic x rays, less than that caused by natural radiation, as shown in Table 14-4. A variety of things can

TABLE 14-3   Occupational carcinogens and industries in which exposure to carcinogens is common

Industrial carcinogens

acrylonitrile, 4-aminodiphenyl, arsenic compounds, asbestos, auramine, benzene, benzidine, benzidine salts, beryllium, bis-(chloromethyl) ether, cadmium compounds, carbon tetrachloride, chloromethyl, chromium compounds, magenta, methyl ether, mustard gas, α-naphthylamine, β-naphthylamine, nickel compounds, oils, soot, tars, vinyl chloride

Industries and occupations

Adhesives, artificial leather, asbestos, asbestos textiles, automobile brakes, biochemical synthesis, burnishing, cement mixing, chemical industry, construction, coal, coke gas, detergent industry, dry battery production, dye making, furniture, glue production, insulation production, petrochemical production, plastics, putty making, rubber industry, shipyards, shoes, water pipe cutters, welding, wood preservation, woodwork be done either to prevent environmental radiation from increasing and to reduce exposure to that which already exists. Clearly, continued atmospheric testing of nuclear bombs will increase the fallout exposure, so that a ban on such tests seems essential. Nuclear power plants produce minor danger, except possibly on a local level. Maintaining a reasonable distance from television sets will reduce x-ray exposure. Of the natural radiations little can be done about cosmic rays, which fall on the earth from the far reaches of the galaxy, and the natural radioactivity of elements in the body. However, exposure to radiation in the soil can be reduced. A government advisory panel, the National Council on Radiation Protection, has estimated that roughly 9000 individuals die each year from lung cancer induced by breathing radon gas. Radon is a naturally occurring radioactive element produced deep within the earth by decay of heavy elements. It slowly rises to the surface and is released into the atmosphere, where its effects are usually minimal. However, radon can enter buildings through cracks in the foundation and flooring. In tightly insulated homes, especially in the colder climates, radon builds up to detectable levels and is breathed in by residents of the house. Simply by opening windows

TABLE 14-4   Annual exposure of humans in the United States to various forms of radiation in 1980

Source	Dose, millirem
Natural radiation	
Cosmic rays	28
Natural radioisotopes in the body	28
Natural radioisotopes in the soil	26
	82
Manmade radiation	
Diagnostic X rays	20
Radioactive drugs	2-4
Consumer products (X rays from TV, radioisotopes in clock dials) and building materials	4-5
Fallout from weapons testing	4-5
Nuclear power plants	<1
	30-35
Total	112-117

Source: National Research Council, Committee on the Biological Effects of Ionizing Radiations. "The Effects on Populations of Exposure to Low Levels of Ionizing Radiation. National Academy Press. 1980.

and doors to exchange the indoor air with outdoor door is probably sufficient to reduce radon buildup, a procedure requiring a certain amount of willpower in the winter in northern parts of the United States, Canada, and Europe. Large buildings are less prone to radon buildup, because by law they have efficient ventilation systems for exchanging air.

Sex and Cancer

Frequent casual sex, especially early in life, is associated with increased risk of cervical cancer in females. The cause is unknown. It has been suggested that some cervical cancers (as well as a few cancers of other types) may be induced by sexually transmitted viruses such as genital herpes. Cleanliness, avoidance of sex with an infected individual, and the use of condoms should reduce the likelihood of transmission of these infectious agents.

Summary

The following actions, based on evidence from animal and/or laboratory studies, and/or human population studies, should help prevent cancers.

1. Stop smoking.
2. Avoid excessive exposure to the sun and other forms of radiation.
3. Avoid exposure to known carcinogens.
4. Avoid heavy consumption of alcohol.
5. Reduce consumption of fats, salt-cured, salt-pickled, smoked, charred, heavily browned, and burned foods.
6. Increase consumption of fruits, vegetables, and whole-grain products, especially those rich in beta-carotene, vitamin A, vitamin C, vitamin E, selenium, and fiber.
7. Drink plenty of water.
8. Avoid frequent sexual contacts with casual partners.

PREVENTING ADVANCED CANCER

The medical profession has been working for years on treatments for cancer, and numerous treatments are effective, including drugs, radiation, radiochemicals, and surgery. However, many of these treatments fail unless the cancer is detected when quite small. There is no doubt that early detection optimizes cure and that it is primarily the responsibility of the individual. For example, cancer can often be prevented completely if premalignant lesions (such as certain sores in the mouth and on the skin) are found before they become cancerous. All individuals must, first, train themselves to become aware of the state of their bodies and changes in the body, and to see a physician, without fear, when any change is noticed. Routine checkups with a variety of standard tests are also essential. These needs are summarized in the list of seven safeguards recommended by the American Cancer Society shown in Table 14-5.

TABLE 14-5   Safeguards urged by the American Cancer Society that could prevent cancer and help prevent advanced cancer

---

The 7 Safeguards

Lung: Don't smoke cigarettes.

Colon-rectum: Get a proctoscope exam as part of a regular checkup after age 40.

Breast: Practice monthly self-examination.

Uterus: Get a Pap smear as part of a regular checkup.

Skin: Avoid overexposure to sunlight.

Oral: Have a regular mouth examination by a physician or dentist.

Complete body: Have an overall physical checkup regularly.

ADDITIONAL READINGS

American Cancer Society. 1983. Cancer Facts and Figures. pp. 1-25.

Ames, B.N. 1983. "Dietary carcinogens and anticarcinogens." Science, 221, 1256.

Ames, B.N. 1984. "Letter on cancer and diet." Science, 192, 658.

Armstrong, B. and R. Doll. 1975. "Environmental factors and cancer incidence and mortality in different countries with special reference to dietary practices." Intern. J. Cancer, 15, 617.

Baltimore, D. 1976. "Viruses, polymerase, and cancer." Science, 192, 632.

Cimino, J.A. (ed.). 1983. Cancer and Environment. Liebert.

Consumers Union. 1983. "Sunscreens." Consumer Reports, 48, 275.

Consumers Union. 1983. "Water filters." Consumer Reports, 48, 68.

DeLuca, L.M. and S.S. Shapiro. 1981. "Modulation of cellular interactions by vitamin A and derivatives (retinoids)." Annals N.Y. Acad. Sci., 359, 1.

Epstein, S.S. and J.B. Swartz. 1984. "Letter on cancer and diet." Science, 224, 658.

Fraumeni, J.F. 1975. Persons at High Risk of Cancer. Academic Press.

Fraumeni, J.F. 1979. "Epidemiological studies of cancer." In Carcinogens: Identification and Mechanisms. A.C. Griffen and C.R. Shawe (eds.). p. 51. Raven.

Griffen, A.C. 1979. "Role of selenium in the chemoprevention of cancer." Adv. Cancer. Res., 29, 419.

Harris, R.H., T. Page, and N.A. Reiches. 1977. "Carcinogenic hazards of organic chemicals in drinking water." Origins of Human Cancer. p. 309.

Henderson, B.E., R.K. Ross, M.C. Pike, and J.T. Casagrande. 1982. "Endogenous hormones as a major factor in human cancer." Cancer Res., 42, 3232.

Hietanen, E. 1980. "Dietary components and cancer." J. Toxicol. Environ. Health, 5-6, 963.

Kallistratos, G. and E. Fasske. 1980. "Inhibition of benzo(a)pyrene carcinogenesis in rats with vitamin C." J. Cancer Res., 97, 91.

Karpas, A. 1982. "Viruses and leukemia." Amer. Scientist, 70, 277.

Kolata, G. 1983. "Does vitamin A prevent cancer?" Science, 223, 1161.

Marx, J.L. 1979. "Low-level radiation: just how bad is it?" Science, 204, 160.

Miller, J.A. 1970. "Carcinogenesis by chemicals." Cancer Res., 30, 559.

National Research Council. "The effects on population of exposure to low levels of ionizing radiation." BEIR Report. p. 91. Washington, D.C.

National Research Council. 1982. Report on Diet, Nutrition, and Cancer.

New York Academy of Sciences. 1977. Cancer and the Worker.

Oppenheimer, S.B. 1983. "Prevention of cancer." Amer. Lab., 15, 66.

Oppenheimer, S.B. 1983. "Control of the spread of cancer." Amer. Clin. Prod. Rev., 2, 12.

Oppenheimer, S.B. 1984. Cancer Prevention Guidebook. Burgess.

Schottenfeld, D. and J.F. Haas. 1979. "Carcinogens in the workplace." Can.-Amer. Cancer J. Clinic., 29, 144.

Sporn, M.B., R.A. Squire, C.C. Brown, and J.M. Smith. 1977. "Retinoic acid: inhibition of bladder carcinogenesis in the rat." Science, 195, 487.

Sporn, M.B., G.R. Prout. 1978. "Retinoid cancer prevention trial begins against bladder cancer." J. Amer. Med. Assoc., 240, 609.

Sporn, M.B. 1980. "Combination chemoprevention of cancer." Nature, 287, 107.

Tomatis, L.C., H. Agthe, H. Bartsch, J. Huff, R. Montesano, E. Saracc, E. Walker, and J. Wilbourn. 1978. "Evaluation of the carcinogenicity of chemicals." Cancer Res., 38, 877.

U.S. Dept. of Health, Education, and Welfare. 1979. Smoking and Health. A Report of the Surgeon General. Washington, D.C.

Wattenberg, L.W. 1978. "Inhibition of chemical carcinogenesis." Adv. Cancer Res., 26, 197.

Wattenberg, L.W. 1981. "Inhibitors of chemical carcinogens." In Cancer: Achievements, Challenges, and Prospects for the 1980's. Vol. 1. Grune and Stratton.

15

Psychosocial Aspects
of Cancer

Few words in the English language bring as much fear to the minds of an individual than cancer. It brings with it a feeling of hopelessness, despair, and finality. Attitudes of friends and family may change when they learn of cancer in an individual, which may compound the fear. Thus, in many ways cancer is a psychological disease. Hundreds of books have been written that deal with these problems, and space is available in this book only to bring out a few of the more salient features. Other psychosocial aspects of cancer include a suspected relation between stress and the probability of developing cancer, and the relation between the cancer patient and his or her physician. These and other topics are the subject of this chapter.

STRESS AND CANCER

Stress contributes to many diseases, for example, heart disease and stroke, though why this is so is rarely clear. In view of the fact that one's emotional state affects the levels of a myriad of hormones and other biological molecules, which exert a wide variety of effects on the body, an effect of stress on the ability of the body to maintain itself in a healthy state comes as no surprise. Probably the most familiar aspects of the effect of emotions on disease are the frequently made observations that depressed people seem to get sick more after than happy people and that patients with a good outlook (the so-called "will to live") have a greater chance of recovery from serious disease. Unfortunately whether the latter is true has never been proved unambiguously.

For several decades many cancer researchers and physicians have suggested that stress is a contributing factor in both the onset and outcome of cancer. Recently, some experimental evidence has shown that emotional, psychosocial, or anxiety-induced stress produces increases concentrations of adrenal corticoid hormones in the blood. Studies with mice indicate that increased concentrations of these hormones reduce the effectiveness and sometimes injure the immune system. Thus, it is possible that stress could leave a person subject to the action of latent viruses, newly formed cancer cells, or any other pathological process normally held in check by the immune system. The experiments with mice will be described.

Two colonies of genetically identical mice of the same age were maintained in separate environments. The mice in one colony lived a relatively stress-free life. The other mice were subjected to various stress-inducing devices, such as occasional spinning. Stressed mice developed increased concentrations of corticosterone in their blood within a few minutes after rotation, and this increase was followed within two hours by visible damage to circulating lymphocytes. In very young mice the thymus gland (which is part of the immune system) actually began to disintegrate within 24 hours. Administrating small amounts of the hormone to unstressed mice simulated these effects. At various times over a period of several months both stressed and unstressed animals were examined for tumors. A variety of tumors, most of which grew rather quickly, were found in the stressed mice, whereas few tumors occurred in the unstressed mice. Administration

of corticosterone to unstressed mice also caused tumor production.
The following interpretation of these experiments has been given.
Stress causes increased levels of the hormone in the blood. High
concentrations of the hormone causes damage to lymphocytes and to
the thymus. Decreased numbers of active circulating T lymphocytes,
which normally are probably able to destroy cancer cells, lead to
enhanced tumor growth. It must be emphasized that such experiments
have not been done on humans (for obvious reasons); also, if such
an effect of stress does occur in humans, only those diseases that
are under partial or complete control of the normal active immune
system would be likely to be brought out of control by stress-induced
impairment of immune function, and this may not be true of all cancers.
Further research on this important topic is in progress.

PERSONALITY TYPES AND CANCER

A controversial topic is whether certain personality types are more
prone to develop cancer and more likely to die of cancer. By
conducting psychological evaluations of cancer patients, several
investigators have found that such individuals often have low-key
personalities and tend to repress outward discharge of emotions.
However, such a characterization may be totally incorrect for a
particular patient, and the findings must be analyzed statistically. At
present, it is thought that increased risk for some cancers may exist
in certain personality types, though the data are not particularly
convincing. In several studies a traumatic personal loss was also
associated with cancer frequency. In one study of adult patients with
lymphoma and leukemia, 30 of 32 women and 16 of 16 men studied
reported a deep personal loss in the previous year. This might simply
be a result of the fact that cancer is a disease of older people, and
older people are more likely to suffer losses among their peers and
loved ones; however, similar results were reported for children with
acute leukemia. Such studies must be interpreted with caution, because
having cancer plays emotional havoc with many individuals and may
have made them exaggerate the importance of the personal losses
reported.

It has often been said that when a person experiences a life-
threatening trauma, the will to live helps the person live and giving
up hastens death. Whereas there is probably some truth to this
statement, solid data have been hard to come by. Several studies
have suggested that individuals who express emotions outwardly, are
angry and clearly are fighting to live, appear to have a better
prognosis than those who give up or consider their situation as
hopeless.

SOCIOLOGICAL ASPECTS OF CANCER

A variety of diseases are less prevalent among the higher socioeconomic
groups. In many cases, this is simply a result of better self care
and higher living standards. Increased survival from many human
diseases among the higher socioeconomic groups is surely due to better
access to health care. Probably an important factor is that people in

the upper groups are more prone to spend their money to see a doctor; thus, tumors are detected in the more favorable early stages.

Sociological factors unrelated to economic status have been associated with the development of cervical cancer. These include early sexual experience, multiple sex partners when young, early marriage, and high incidence of marital problems. At one time premarital sex and multiple partners were more prevalent among the lower socioeconomic groups, but this is no longer the case.

EMOTIONAL RESPONSE TO THE DIAGNOSIS OF CANCER

As mentioned in the introduction, a positive diagnosis of cancer is a fearful thing to most people. Whereas the prognosis for some cancers is poor, for most cancers treatment is sufficiently effective that such fear is unnecessary. The fear is clearly associated with the knowledge that cancer often leads to death. However, having a heart attack and surviving does not usually produce an emotional response of such depth.

When a person is first told that he or she has cancer, the usual response is immediate horror followed by denial: a mistake has been made. When assured that the cancer is real and that it can be treated, a typical patient becomes somewhat calmer for the duration of the visit with the doctor, but this apparent calm is short-lived. Over the next few days many patients experience what could be called a reevaluation of life. As an example, consider what was stated by one patient. This patient is an interesting case because the feeling to be described came before the biopsy, which proved to be negative (that is, there was no cancer). "When told that I probably had lung cancer, I was immediately plunged into a severe depression, even though I knew that the diagnosis was not yet certain. After leaving the doctor, I could not shake the feeling that I would be dead within a year, even though I had been told that the suspected tumor was very small and the type of cancer had quite a high 5-year survival level. While driving home, my thoughts switched back and forth between concern for my teenage children and how I would spend my remaining year. I had been working quite hard in the previous weeks, and suddenly it all seemed to be pointless. I felt that I should spend all of my time enjoying life. I thought that if, on the other hand, I worked even harder, I could provide my children with more money to live on when I died. I decided to devote my entire remaining life to assuring the security of my children. When reaching my house, I looked around and decided that I had to start going through all of my things and throwing away what was no longer needed. I wanted to go over all of my finances, so my children would know exactly what they had and what they had to do. I realized that my children didn't know how to use certain household appliances (like the washing machine) and many useful tools, so I had better teach them these things right away. Clearly, within two hours of being told that I <u>might</u> have cancer, I was preparing for my death. I then agonized over whether I should tell them or anyone else. I decided not to do so, for fear of worrying everyone. Rationally, I knew that I might not even have the cancer, but I had the urge to talk to people about it. I did not do so and carried the awful burden alone for one week. A visit to a psychotherapist made me look at things more realistically and armed me for the week while I was waiting for the biopsy result. However, during this time I found that only hard work and total distract could keep my mind off of my death. I had many discussions with myself in which I tried to imagine what the world and my house would be like without me. I finally talked to a friend who suggested that I have optimistic fantasies. So, I rehearsed my coming meeting with the doctor, hearing him tell me that the biopsy was negative. At some moments I could convince myself that I was predicting the correct outcome. At other moments, I knew I was wrong. There was no doubt in my mind that I was going through the most awful experience of my life. Interestingly, when I finally was told by the doctor that I did not have cancer, my reaction was not one of relief, for in fact, I had convinced myself that this was to be the outcome. Since this terrible time I have often reviewed my thoughts and tried to understand the magnitude of my fear. I have not succeeded though."

Notice in this quotation the early feeling of helplessness and hopelessness and the undercurrent of setting one's affairs in order. These are common emotions with the cancer patient. However, even the soldier entering battle does not usually do so with such feelings of despair. What in our society is the source of the magnitude of this fear? It is difficult to say, but there are many possibilities. One is certainly that one hears of death by cancer at a very early age. Since everyone ultimately dies and since cancer is to a great extent a disease of the elderly, one learns to associate it with death. Thus, even when one is given a diagnosis of skin cancer, with its nearly 100% survival, one gets depressed; the message is cancer, pain, death, not treatment and high frequency of survival. To a great extent, the survival statistics have been interpreted with the wrong psychology. Consider a cancer in which the 5-year survival is 70%. One can say, "I have a 30% chance of being dead within 5 years (the pessimistic approach)," or "I have a 70% chance of being alive in 5 years (the optimistic approach)." Clearly, the second attitude is more realistic, more profitable, and will give one a better life; however, the former attitude is often the more prevalent one.

Another example from statistics is the following. Patients with certain types of breast cancer with minimal involvement of local lymph nodes have a 5-year survival of about 65% without chemotherapy. One patient, an attractive woman who had just had a breast removed, was told that this survival level could be increased to about 95% with a drug regimen that would make her feel fairly bad for some months and would make her lose her hair. Her first reaction was that it would not be worth it. She felt that the probability of her survival was only 95/65 or about 50% greater and she would be losing out on a good year (the first) of her remaining five years. Note that she, like the person quoted above, was planning for her death. She changed her mind when it was suggested that she think about the statistics in a different way. With a 65% survival level, she had a 35% chance of dying within 5 years. With therapy the chance of her being dead was now 100 - 95 = 5%, a 35/5 = 7-fold lower chance of dying. This was in 1975; she viewed the situation optimistically, opted for treatment, and remains alive and healthy, enjoying life.

Unfortunately, family and friends often react to a diagnosis of cancer with the same sinking feeling experienced by the patient. This attitude is sensed by the patient, who feels even more remorseful. It makes sense that family members should relate to the patient with the goal of helping the individual fight the damaging psychological aspects of the disease. The will to live and to respond favorably to treatment should be strengthened, and this is aided when family members support the patient and relate to the patient in a positive, loving manner. As indicated earlier in the text, cancer is the most curable of the killer diseases, and all patients should be made to feel that they are loved, that their treatment is helping them, and that a concerted effort of personal support is behind them all the way. Treating patients with respect and concern can only help them respond favorably to treatment. Even in cases in which little hope for cure exists, respect and concern will go a long way in helping patients deal with their disease.

People involved in health care can contribute significantly to the psychological well-being of the cancer patient. It is the responsibility of physicians, nurses, and all medical personnel to treat the patient with concern and respect. If family members are given the time to understand the diagnosis and are given some hope for successful treatment, they will be far better able to help the patient form a positive outlook that could go a long way in improving the prognosis of an individual's disease. Even when an individual is close to death, close personal relationships and respect will give both the patient and family added comfort and support. Family members who are close to patients during the final days and relate well to the patients during these times are more likely to be able to cope with the loved one's death and are more likely to be free of the guilt and regret that may accompany such a death.

PSYCHOLOGICAL RESPONSE TO SURGERY

Patients who have been treated for cancer by surgery often feel that they are disfigured and will lose the love of family members and friends. This is especially true of women who have had a mastectomy (removal of a breast) and fear that they may have lost their husband's love. The self image of such a patient is often poor, and this is reflected in many aspects of the individual's life. It is therefore important that such individuals be treated with dignity and respect and that family members and friends are counseled to relate to them with the same respect and understanding as they did before the surgery. The American Cancer Society, for example, offers a Reach to Recovery program for mastectomy patients that is run by trained volunteers who themselves have had a mastectomy. This program offers preoperative and postoperative discussions that are very supportive of the patients. Colostomy patients (who have had their bowels removed and who excrete into a bag attached to the lower abdomen) also benefit greatly from the preoperative and postoperative discussions with individuals that have had similar operations and have returned to a full social life. Health professionals and volunteers, together with a patient's family, can offer the patient real support and understanding so that he/she may return to a full and enjoyable life. With proper support they can come to realize that a colostomy is an inconvenience rather than a deformity.

The references given at the end of this chapter explore the topic of psychosocial aspects of cancer in far greater depth than the brief introductory treatment given in this text. Especially recommended for the family with a terminal cancer patient is the book by Kübler-Ross, who documented the course of her own death as a process with dignity.

HEALTH CARE FOR CANCER PATIENTS

All doctors do not have the same qualifications, neither in knowledge, experience, human understanding, nor compassion. Similarly, all hospitals do not have the same facilities. In this section, we point out what should be looked for when selecting a doctor and a hospital for cancer treatment. These selections should not be made casually and should be a result of rational consideration rather than chance, rumor, or friendship.

Choosing a Physician

The following are frequent characteristics of physicians who are found to be most helpful and competent.

1. Physicians who practice in large groups such as in hospitals and multispecialty groups are usually subject to constant interactions with and review by their peers.
2. Physicians who practice as part of a university or medical school, hospital, or a large community hospital interact with many experts and keep abreast of the latest research. They also deal with large numbers of patients and are likely to have more experience in treating specific cancers than physicians who see few patients.
3. Physicians who are board-certified by experts in their specialty area have passed rigorous examinations in their specialties. Cancer treatment, or oncology, is a recognized specialty, and such specialists are highly qualified to treat both common and rare cancers. The Directory of Medical Specialists, available at most libraries, lists those physicians who are board certified. Local or state medical societies and health departments may also be able to supply information regarding board certification of specific physicians.
4. Physicians who explain things clearly, are easy to communicate with, keep complete and accurate records, have all information about a case available when communicating with patients, and are friendly and concerned usually provide patients with a feeling of well-being. A good relationship with a physician often means a better response to treatment.
5. Physicians should encourage second opinions if a patient wishes them. Doctors who frown on additional consultation may be insecure, incompetent, or both; they are often

concerned with their own egos rather than the well being of the patient. Individuals can contact the nearest cancer center (see Appendix), the American Cancer Society, the Directory of Medical Specialists, or the National Cancer Institute for the names of superior specialists who can give second opinions. The National Cancer Institute and many cancer centers have toll free phone numbers for use by the public. These are listed in the Appendix.

Hospitals

Because of the huge number of cancer patients in the United States, the U.S. government, state governments, and numerous cancer societies engage in evaluation of hospitals with respect to their ability to treat cancer patients. Following is information that individuals should know in selecting a hospital for treatment of cancer. It should be realized that all doctors are not able to practice at all hospitals, so a choice of hospital may limit the choice of a doctor.

1. About 1600 hospitals in the United States lack minimum accreditation by the Joint Commission on Accreditation of Hospitals. Such accreditation is a minimum standard that assures adequate care. The large number of hospitals that lack accreditation is reason enough for an individual to make a few inquiries before being admitted to a hospital for the treatment of any disease including cancer.

2. Comprehensive Cancer Centers are facilities designated by the National Cancer Institute as major regional centers for cancer study, care, and training. They are among the most up-to-date of cancer-care institutions. There is only a small number of such centers in the United States. Such centers provide information and consultation to many individuals and physicians not necessarily affiliated with the centers. People living near one of these centers may wish to take advantage of the information, consultation, or care provided by these facilities. Clinical cancer centers are also designated and supported by the National Cancer Institute and provide many of the same up-to-date services as the comprehensive cancer centers.

3. All hospitals accredited by the Joint Commission on Accreditation of Hospitals should provide adequate care. Hospitals with residency and/or internship programs can probably give even better care. Teaching hospitals affiliated with medical schools usually provide excellent care, because they attract top physicians as faculty members of the medical schools. Hospitals with cancer programs approved by the American College of Surgeons have multidisciplinary cancer committees and other requirements that help assure excellent care.

4. A large hospital is, on the average, better than a very small hospital. Large hospitals admit many patients, and physicians

in these hospitals get more experience in treating a variety of diseases. Larger hospitals also often have more extensive facilities for modern care. Some studies suggest that very small hospitals (less than 100 beds) may have significantly higher death rates than larger hospitals. Most physicians can admit patients to more than one hospital. Thus, if a patient is not satisfied with the choice of hospital made by his/her physician, the matter should be discussed with the doctor, so that an alternative arrangement can be made.

ADDITIONAL READINGS

Edlin, G. and E. Golanty. 1985. Health and Wellness. 2nd ed. Chapters 10, 17, and 24. Jones and Bartlett.

Fuller, B.F. and E. Fuller. 1978. Physician or Magician. The Myths and Realities of Patient Care. McGraw-Hill.

Higginson, J. 1976. "A hazardous society? Individual versus community responsibility in cancer prevention." Amer. J. Public Health, 66, 359.

Holland, J. F. 1969. "Prediction of time of death in patients with advanced cancer." Ann. N.Y. Acad. Sci., 164, 678.

Kübler-Ross, E. 1974. Questions and Answers on Death and Dying. Macmillan.

LeShan, L. 1966. "An emotional life-history pattern associated with neoplastic disease." Ann. N.Y. Acad. Sci., 125, 790.

Markel, W.M., and V.B. Sinon. 1978. "The hospice concept." CA, A Cancer Journal for Clinicians., 28, 225.

Morra, M., and Potts, E. 1980. Choices. Realistic Alternatives in Cancer treatment. Avon.

Simonton, O.C., S.S. Simonton, and J. Creighton. 1978. Getting Well Again. Tarcher.

Weisman, A. 1979. Coping with Cancer. McGraw-Hill.

Winick, M. 1977. Nutrition and Cancer. Wiley.

The American Cancer Society, local cancer societies, and local clinics and health services provide pamphlets on the psychological aspects of cancer.

16

The Prognosis
for Cancer

What areas offer most hope for improving the prognosis for the various forms of cancer? Improved diagnostic techniques are a very realistic possibility in the near future. Throughout this text, we have stressed that the prognosis of cancers that have not yet spread is often very good. Early diagnosis is crucial in identifying cancers before spread to secondary sites has occurred. Improved x-ray technology, immunological tests for cancer antigens, and other biochemical diagnostic tests may help identify cancers at much earlier stages than is now possible. To have to wait until a lung cancer consists of over one billion cells is a major reason for treatment failure in this disease. A tumor of such a size may have been 10 years in the making and 10 years in a stage that currently cannot be diagnosed and in which there was ample time to spread. Like many other cancers that can be diagnosed early, lung cancer should be much more easily cured if early diagnosis can be accomplished.

Some say that if everyone stopped smoking, eventually 50 percent of all cancer deaths would be eliminated. Not only lung cancer, but cancer of the upper respiratory passages, upper digestive tract, bladder, mouth, lips, and tongue, to name a few, are most frequent in smokers. The incidence of some cancers is even higher among people who are exposed to the smoke of others, for example, children in a smoking household and people working in smoky rooms. Recent studies suggest that low-tar, low-nicotine cigarettes are reducing lung cancer rates in smokers, so there is some reason for optimism. It is mind-boggling to imagine that one single step, elimination of smoking, could do more to eliminate cancer than the billions of dollars spent on cancer research, treatment, and the like. Continued mass media education, hopefully, will keep pressure on industry to make safer cigarettes and, more important, on people to stop smoking. What is true of cigarettes is also true of numerous other carcinogens. Industry must be made to reduce the levels of hazardous agents in the environment, and people must be on constant vigil to be sure that their representatives in the government are doing their jobs in this important area. If only there were substantial profit to industry in eliminating all suspect agents, we would not have to depend on government regulation. However, we should not blame industry for all our woes, because death rates for many cancers do not seem to have increased in the last thirty years, whereas industrial production of plastics, synthetic rubber, pesticides, etc., has increased more than 100-fold.

The relation between diet and cancer risk is an exciting area that is just beginning to yield solid data. For example, increased intake of fiber and decreased intake of certain fats over a long period of time may substantially reduce the risk of some cancers. Although the habits of Americans may be hard to change, continued studies in this area may yield information that the public will find difficult to dismiss.

New approaches in cancer treatment are making the future for cancer patients brighter. Chemotherapy has apparently cured numerous leukemia cases that not too long ago were invariably fatal. Immunotherapy is coming of age and becoming more than just an experimental form of cancer treatment. Radiotherapy with some new forms of particle radiation may permit near total destruction of deep tumors with little damage to surrounding normal tissue. Whether or not major advances in treating metastatic cancers will occur in the near future will probably depend on the development of chemotherapeutic or immunotherapeutic protocols that are specific for destroying cancer cells with little damage to normal tissues.

Most of the promising approaches just mentioned have already, in part, been developed and are beginning to provide improved prognoses for some forms of cancer. However, the total elimination of cancer will probably require a better understanding of cancer at the cellular level. The molecular nature of the factors involved in gene expression, mutation, and carcinogenesis are not well understood. If indeed there is a single key defect in cancer cells, understanding of this defect may lead to prevention and cure of the disease. If, on the other hand, numerous cellular mechanisms are vulnerable to alterations that could induce cancer, general prevention and cure of the disease may be unrealistic goals for the near future. The discovery of oncogenes is an important step forward in understanding details of the process of cancer induction.

We know that the essential feature of cancer cells is their continuous, unregulated growth, and no other single characteristic is common to all cancers. If growth control in all cells is regulated by a single key mechanism, such as some particular gene or set of genes, and if the means by which growth is controlled in cells becomes understood, it is likely that a truly effective means of controlling cancer may be developed. Numerous attempts at controlling the growth of cancer cells have already been made. Protease inhibitors, metabolic inhibitors, compounds that bind to cell surface carbohydrates, and proteins that help the body fight virus infections are a few of the agents that have been used to prevent cancer cells from growing in an unregulated manner. To date, no single agent has successfully inhibited the growth of all cancer cells.

Some investigators are attempting to control cancer cells by developing vaccines that stimulate the immune system generally and/or specifically. General immunostimulants include BCG, while specific agents include vaccines made with live or killed cancer cells or cancer cell surface antigens. Unfortunately, all or even most cancer cells do not share similar cell surface antigens that are specific for cancer cells. Thus, it is unlikely that a vaccine against all or most cancers could be produced in the same way as has been successfully accomplished for the many infectious diseases, such as smallpox, polio, and diphtheria. However, immunotherapy is promising because of the potential specificity in killing only cancer cells, and major efforts in this area are underway; some are now showing limited success.

The future will also probably bring increased awareness on the part of individuals with respect to habits and agents that increase cancer risk. Behavioral changes on the part of individuals of habits and lifestyle may play an increasingly important role in decreasing cancer risk.

I believe that this nation and the world must support basic research in science even if it does not appear to be directly relevant to human benefit. The cures to many diseases have often resulted from information gleaned from totally unrelated areas over a period of decades. For example, work on the nature of gene regulation in bacteria or fruit flies might well lead to an understanding of defective growth control in cancer cells. Work in very simple, primitive systems often leads to a better understanding of how human cells work. The point is that the functioning of an organism with a few dozen genes is usually more easily understood than that of a cell with thousands of genes. Thus, cancer research should be thought of as basic research, and any system that promises to reveal some basic information about cells may lead to a key in the cancer puzzle. The successful elimination of cancer will probably result from basic scientific research by good people in all fields, and such work must be vigorously supported. Short-sighted attempts to cure cancer in a given time period will probably fail. Prevention and cure of most cancers will occur with time if scientists are allowed to pursue basic information freely and with wholehearted support. Cancer research and other areas of basic research, such as those dealing with growth control, differentiation, and gene regulation, are inextricably intertwined.

Cancer prevention will certainly receive more attention in the future as indicated at recent annual meetings of the American Association for Cancer Research. A persistent message at this meetings is that cancer can be treated, but, more importantly, can be avoided.

ADDITIONAL READINGS

American Cancer Society. 1977. "Lung cancer and smoking." Cancer Facts and Figures. American Cancer Society.

American Cancer Society. 1980. Cancer Facts and Figures. American Cancer Society.

Hodgson, T. A. 1975. "The economic costs of cancer." In D. Schottenfeld, ed., Cancer Epidemiology and Prevention: Current Concepts. C.C. Thomas.

Wynder, E. L., and Hoffmann, D. 1975. "The tenth anniversary of the surgeon general's report on smoking and health. Have we made any progress?" J. Natl. Cancer Inst., 54, 533.

Appendix: Cancer Information Services

The following listings offer cancer information to the public. Some of the listings may change over time and should be verified by contacting the appropriate agency for the most recent information.

CANCER INFORMATION SERVICES

The National Cancer Institute of the United States Public Health Service maintains the Cancer Information Service by which people anywhere in the United States can telephone to obtain information about cancer.

From most locations dialing the toll-free number 1-800-4-CANCER will connect you automatically with the regional office service your area. Spanish-speaking staff members are available (simply by asking in Spanish) from the following areas: California (area codes 213, 619, 714, and 805), Florida, Georgia, Illinois, Northern New Jersey, New York City, and Texas.

Only three locations cannot use the above toll-free number. The numbers for these locations are as follows: Alaska: 1-800-638-6070. Hawaii: Oahu, 808-524-1234; neighbor islands can call collect. Washington, D.C. (and Maryland and Virginia suburbs: 202-636-5700.

The National Cancer Institute also publishes a monthly list of publications available free of charge. To obtain the list, write:

> Office of Cancer Communications
> National Cancer Institute, Bldg. 31, Room 10A18
> Bethesda, MD 20205.

AMERICAN CANCER SOCIETY

The American Cancer Society provides the public with information about cancer. The national office is located at: American Cancer Society, 777 Third Avenue, New York, New York 10017. Mailing addresses and telephone numbers of the various regional offices follow:

Alabama Division, Inc.
402 Office Park
Suite 300
Birmingham, AL 352223
205-879-2242

Alaska Division, Inc.
1343 G Street
Anchorage, AK 9950I
907-277-8690

Arizona Division, Inc.
634 West Indian School Road
P.O. Box 33187
Phoenix, AZ 85067
602-234-3266

Arkansas Division, Inc.
5520 West Markham Street
P.O. Box 3822
Little Rock, AR 72203
501-664-3480-1-2

California Division, Inc.
1710 Webster Street
Oakland, CA 94604
415-777-1800

Colorado Division, Inc.
2255 S. Oneida
P.O. Box 18268
Denver, CO 80218
303-758-2030

Connecticut Division, Inc.
Barnes Park South
14 Village Lane
Wallingford, CT 06492
203-265-7161

Delaware Division, Inc.
1708 Lovering Avenue
Wilmington, DE 19806
302-654-6267

Dist. of Columbia Division, Inc.
Universal Building, South
1825 Connecticut Ave. N.W.
Washington, D.C. 20009
202-483-2600

Florida Division, Inc.
1001 South MacDill Avenue
Tampa, FL 33609
813-253-0541

Georgia Division, Inc.
1422 W. Peachtree Road, NW
Atlanta, GA 30309
404-892-0026

Hawaii Division, Inc.
Community Services Center Bldg.
200 North Vineyard Blvd.
Honolulu, HI 96817
808-531-1662-3-4-5

Idaho Division, Inc.
1609 Abbs Street
P.O. Box 5386
Boise, ID 83705
208-343-4609

Illinois Division, Inc.
37 South Wabash Avenue
Chicago, IL 60603
312-372-0472

Indiana Division, Inc.
9575 N. Valparaiso
Indianapolis, IN 46268
317-872-4432

Iowa Division, Inc.
Highway No. 18 West
P.O. Box 980
Mason City, IA 50401
515-423-0712

Kansas Division, Inc.
3003 Van Buren Street
Topeka, KS 66611
913-267-0131

Kentucky Division, Inc.
Medical Arts Bldg.
1169 Eastern Parkway
Louisville, KY 40217
502-459-1867

Louisiana Division, Inc.
Masonic Temple Bldg., Room 810
333 St. Charles Avenue
New Orleans, LA 70130
504-523-2029

Maine Division, Inc.
Federal and Green Streets
Brunswick, ME 04011
207-729-3339

Maryland Division, Inc.
1840 York Road
Timonium, MD 21093
301-561-4790

Massachusetts Division, Inc.
247 Commonwealth Avenue
Boston, MA 02116
617-267-2650

Michigan Division, Inc.
1205 East Saginaw Street
Lansing, MI 48906
517-371-2920

Minnesota Division, Inc.
2750 Park Avenue
Minneapolis, MN 55407
612-871-2111

Mississippi Division, Inc.
345 North Mart Plaza
Jackson, MS 39206
601-362-8874

Missouri Division, Inc.
332 American Ave., Box 1066
Jefferson City, MO 65101
314-636-3195

Montana Division, Inc.
2820 First Avenue South
Billings, MT 59101
406-252-7111

Nebraska Division, Inc.
8502 W. Center Rd.
Omaha, NE 68124
402-551-2422

Nevada Division, Inc.
1325 E. Harmon
Las Vegas, NV 89109
702-798-6877

New Hampshire Division, Inc.
686 Mast Rd
Manchester, NH 03102
603-669-3270

New Jersey Division, Inc.
CN2201, 2600 Route 1
North Brunswick, NJ 08902
201-297-8000

New Mexico Division, Inc.
5800 Lomas Blvd. N.E.
Albuquerque, NM 87110
505-262-2336

New York State Division, Inc.
6725 Lyons Street
P.O. Box 7
East Syracuse, NY 13057
315-437-7025

Long Island Division, Inc.
535 Broad Hollow Road
Melville, NY 11746
516-420-1111

New York City Division, Inc.
19 West 56th Street
New York, NY 10019
212-586-8700

Queens Division, Inc.
116-25 Queens Boulevard
Forest Hills, NY 11375
212-263-2224

Westchester Division, Inc.
901 North Broadway
White Plains, NY 10603
914-949-4800

North Carolina Division, Inc.
11 S. Boylan
Suite 221
Raleigh, NC 27603
919-834-8463

North Dakota Division, Inc.
115 Roberts Street
Hotel Graver Annex Bldg.
P.O. Box 426
Fargo, ND 58102
701-232-1385

Ohio Division, Inc.
1375 Euclid Ave.
Suite 312
Cleveland, OH 44115
216-771-6700

Oklahoma Division, Inc.
3800 North Cromwell
Oklahoma City, OK 73112
405-946-5000

Oregon Division, Inc.
0330 SW Curry
Portland, OR 97201
503-295-6422

Pennsylvania Division, Inc.
Rte 422 and Sipe Ave.
P.O. Box 416
Hershey, PA 17111
717-533-6144

    Philadelphia Division, Inc.
    1422 Chestnut Street
    Philadelphia, PA 19102
    215-665-2900

Puerto Rico Division, Inc.
Avenue Domenech 273
Hato Rey, P.R.)
GPO Box 6004
San Juan, PR 00936
809-764-2295

Rhode Island Division, Inc.
345 Blackstone Blvd.
Providence, RI 02906
401-831-6970

South Carolina Division, Inc.
2442 Devine Street
Columbia, SC 29205
803-256-0245

South Dakota Division, Inc.
1025 N. Minnesota Ave.
Sioux Falls, SD 57104
605-336-0897

Tennessee Division, Inc.
7131 Melpark Dr.
Nashville, TN 37204
615-383-1710

Texas Division, Inc.
3834 Spicewood Springs Road
P.O. Box 9863
Austin, TX 78766
512-345-4560

Utah Division, Inc.
610 East South Temple
Salt Lake City, UT 84102
801-322-0431

Vermont Division, Inc.
13 Loomis Street, Drawer C
Montpelier, VT 05602
802-223-2348

Virginia Division, Inc.
4240 Park Place Ct., Box 1547
Glen Allen, VA 23060
804-270-0142

Washington Division, Inc.
120 First Avenue N
Seattle, WA 98109
206-283-1152

West Virginia Division, Inc.
240 Capitol Street, Suite 100
Charleston, WV 25301
304-344-3611

Wisconsin Division, Inc.
615 North Sherman Ave., Box 1626
Madison, WI 53701
608-294-0487

    Milwaukee Division, Inc.
    11401 W. Watertown Plank Rd.
    Wawatosa, WI 53226
    414-453-4500

Wyoming Division, Inc.
Indian Hills Center
506 Shoshoni
Cheyenne, WY 82009
307-638-3331

Affiliate of the
American Cancer Society
Canal Zone Cancer Committee
Drawer A
Balboa Heights, Canal Zone

COMPREHENSIVE CANCER CENTERS DESIGNATED BY THE NATIONAL CANCER INSTITUTE

These centers, which have met rigorously criteria imposed by the National Cancer Advisory Board, offer up-to-date information and treatment of cancer.

ALABAMA

Comprehensive Cancer Center
Univ. of Alabama
Lurleen Wallace Tumor Institute
1824 6th Ave. South
Birmingham, AL 35294
205-934-5077

CALIFORNIA

Univ. of Southern California
Comprehensive Cancer Center
1441 Eastlake Avenue
Los Angeles, CA 90033
213-224-6416

UCLA-Jonsson Comprehensive
   Cancer Center
Louis Factor Health Sciences Bldg.
10833 LeConte Ave.
Los Angeles, CA 90024
213-825-5268

CONNECTICUT

Yale University
Comprehensive Cancer Center
333 Cedar Street
New Haven, CT 06510
203-785-4095

DISTRICT OF COLUMBIA

Vincent T. Lombardi Cancer
   Research Center
Georgetown University
3800 Reservoir Road, N.W.
Washington, DC 20007
202-625-7721

Howard University
   Cancer Research Center
Department of Oncology
2041 Georgia Avenue, N.W.
Washington, DC 20060
200-636-7697

FLORIDA

Comprehensive Cancer Center
   for the State of Florida
Univ. of Miami School of Medicine
1475 N.W. 12th Ave.
Miami, FL 33101
305-545-7707

ILLINOIS

Illinois Cancer Council
36 S. Wabash Avenue
Chicago, IL 60603
312-346-9813

MARYLAND

Johns Hopkins University
Comprehensive Cancer Center
600 N. Wolfe Street
Baltimore, MD 21205
301-955-8822

MASSACHUSETTS

Dana-Farber Cancer Institute
44 Binney Street
Boston, MA 02115
617-732-3555

MICHIGAN

Michigan Cancer Foundation
Meyer Prentis Cancer Center
110 East Warren Street
Detroit, MI 48201
313-833-0710

MINNESOTA

Mayo Clinic
200 First Street, S.W.
Rochester, MN 55905
507-284-8964

NEW YORK

Columbia University Cancer
   Research Center
701 West 168th Street
New York, NY 10032
212-694-3647

Memorial Sloan-Kettering
   Cancer Center
1275 York Avenue
New York, NY 10021
212-794-6561

Roswell Park Memorial Institute
666 Elm Street
Buffalo, NY 14263
716-845-5770

NORTH CAROLINA

Duke Comprehensive Cancer
   Center
P.O. Box 3814
Duke Univ. Medical Center
Durham, NC 27710
919-684-2282

OHIO

Ohio State Univ. Comprehensive
   Cancer Center
410 W. 12th Ave.
Columbus, OH 43210
614-422-5022

PENNSYLVANIA

Fox Chase Cancer Center
7701 Burholme Avenue
Philadelphia, PA 19111
215-728-2781

Univ. of Pennsylvania
   Cancer Center
3400 Spruce St.
7th Floor, Silverstein Pavilion
Philadelphia, PA 19104
215-662-3910

TEXAS

University of Texas System
   Cancer Center
M.D. Anderson Hospital and
   Tumor Institute
6723 Bertner Avenue
Houston, TX 77030
713-792-6000

WASHINGTON

Fred Hutchinson Cancer
   Research Center
1124 Columbia Street
Seattle, WA 98104
206-292-2930

WISCONSIN

Wisconsin Clinical Cancer
   Center
University of Wisconsin
Dept of Human Oncology
600 Highland Avenue
Madison, WI 53792
608-263-8610

CANCER TREATMENT CENTERS APPROVED BY THE AMERICAN COLLEGE OF SURGEONS

All hospitals and medical centers are not accredited by the American College of Surgeons as cancer treatment centers. To aid a potential cancer patient in selecting a hospital or to give a patient and his/her family confidence in the hospital by the physician, all of the approved centers are listed below. This includes a large number of hospitals and is taken from the book Cancer Programs Approved, issued by the Commission on Cancer of the American College of Surgeons. Because of the great length of the list, the original computer printout of this book has been reprinted. To obtain more up-to-late listings, contact: Assistant Director, Professional Activities (Cancer), American College of Surgeons, 55 E. Erie St., Chicago, IL 60611.

City	State	Hospital
AL	BIRMINGHAM	BAPTIST MED CNTR - PRINCETON
AL	BIRMINGHAM	BROOKWOOD MEDICAL CENTER
AL	BIRMINGHAM	CARRAWAY METHODIST MED CNTR
AL	BIRMINGHAM	UNIV OF ALABAMA HOSPITALS
AL	BIRMINGHAM	VETERANS ADMIN MED CNTR
AL	GADSDEN	BAPTIST MEMORIAL HOSPITAL
AL	MOBILE	MOBILE INFIRMARY
AL	MOBILE	UNIV OF SOUTH ALABAMA MED CNTR
AL	TUSKEGEE	VETERANS ADMIN MED CNTR
AR	FAYETTEVILLE	WASHINGTON REGIONAL MED CNTR
AR	FORT SMITH	SPARKS REGIONAL MEDICAL CENTER
AR	FORT SMITH	ST EDWARD MERCY MEDICAL CENTER
AR	LITTLE ROCK	VETERANS ADMIN MED CNTR
AR	ROGERS	ST MARY-ROGERS MEML HOSP
AZ	FLAGSTAFF	FLAGSTAFF MEDICAL CENTER
AZ	MESA	DESERT SAMARITAN HOSPITAL
AZ	MESA	MESA LUTHERAN HOSPITAL
AZ	PHOENIX	GOOD SAMARITAN MEDICAL CENTER
AZ	PHOENIX	MARICOPA MEDICAL CENTER
AZ	PHOENIX	PHOENIX MEMORIAL HOSPITAL
AZ	PHOENIX	VETERANS ADMIN MED CNTR
AZ	SCOTTSDALE	SCOTTSDALE MEMORIAL HOSPITAL
AZ	TUCSON	TUCSON MEDICAL CENTER
AZ	TUCSON	UNIVERSITY HOSPITAL
CA	ALHAMBRA	ALHAMBRA COMMUNITY HOSPITAL
CA	ANAHEIM	ANAHEIM MEMORIAL HOSPITAL
CA	ANAHEIM	HUMANA HOSPITAL WEST ANAHEIM
CA	ANAHEIM	MARTIN LUTHER HOSP MED CNTR
CA	APPLE VALLEY	ST MARY DESERT VALLEY HOSPITAL
CA	ARCADIA	METHODIST HOSP OF SOUTH CALIF
CA	BAKERSFIELD	KERN MEDICAL CENTER
CA	BAKERSFIELD	SAN JOAQUIN COMMUNITY HOSPITAL
CA	BELLFLOWER	BELLWOOD GENERAL HOSPITAL
CA	BELLFLOWER	KAISER FDN HOSP (ROS)
CA	BERKELEY	ALTA BATES HOSPITAL
CA	BERKELEY	HERRICK HOSPITAL & HLTH CENTER
CA	BUENA PARK	LA PALMA INTERCOMMUNITY HOSP
CA	BURBANK	ST JOSEPH MEDICAL CENTER
CA	BURLINGAME	PENINSULA HOSPITAL & MED CNTR
CA	CANOGA PARK	WEST HILLS MEDICAL CENTER
CA	CASTRO VALLEY	EDEN HOSPITAL
CA	CHICO	N T ENLOE MEMORIAL HOSPITAL

City	State	Hospital
CA	CONCORD	MT DIABLO HOSPITAL MED CNTR
CA	COVINA	INTER-COMMUNITY MEDICAL CENTER
CA	DOWNEY	DOWNEY COMMUNITY HOSPITAL
CA	DUARTE	CITY OF HOPE NATL MED CNTR
CA	DUARTE	SANTA TERESITA HOSPITAL
CA	ESCONDIDO	PALOMAR MEMORIAL HOSPITAL
CA	FONTANA	KAISER FDN HOSP (SIE)
CA	FOUNTAIN VALLEY	FOUNTAIN VALLEY COMM HOSPITAL
CA	FRESNO	FRESNO COMMUNITY HOSP MED CNTR
CA	FRESNO	VALLEY CHILDREN'S HOSPITAL
CA	FRESNO	VETERANS ADMIN MED CNTR
CA	FULLERTON	ST JUDE HOSP & REHAB CENTER
CA	GLENDALE	GLENDALE ADVENTIST MED CNTR
CA	GLENDALE	MEMORIAL HOSPITAL OF GLENDALE
CA	GLENDORA	FOOTHILL PRESBYTERIAN HOSPITAL
CA	GLENDORA	GLENDORA COMMUNITY HOSPITAL
CA	GRANADA HILLS	GRANADA HILLS COMM HOSPITAL
CA	HARBOR CITY	BAY HARBOR HOSPITAL
CA	HARBOR CITY	KAISER FDN HOSP (VER)
CA	HAWTHORNE	ROBERT F. KENNEDY MED CENTER
CA	HUNTINGTON BEACH	PACIFICA COMMUNITY HOSPITAL
CA	IMOLA	NAPA STATE HOSPITAL
CA	INDIO	INDIO COMMUNITY HOSPITAL
CA	INGLEWOOD	CENTINELA HOSPITAL MED CNTR
CA	INGLEWOOD	DANIEL FREEMAN MEM HOSPITAL
CA	LA JOLLA	GREEN HOSP OF SCRIPPS CLINIC
CA	LA JOLLA	SCRIPPS MEMORIAL HOSPITAL
CA	LA MESA	GROSSMONT DISTRICT HOSPITAL
CA	LAGUNA HILLS	SADDLEBACK COMMUNITY HOSPITAL
CA	LIVERMORE	VETERANS ADMIN MED CNTR
CA	LOMA LINDA	LOMA LINDA UNIVERSITY MED CNTR
CA	LONG BEACH	LONG BEACH COMMUNITY HOSPITAL
CA	LONG BEACH	LOS ALTOS HOSPITAL
CA	LONG BEACH	MEMORIAL HOSPITAL MED CNTR
CA	LONG BEACH	ST MARY MEDICAL CENTER
CA	LONG BEACH	VETERANS ADMIN MED CNTR
CA	LOS ALAMITOS	LOS ALAMITOS MEDICAL CENTER
CA	LOS ANGELES	CALIFORNIA HOSPITAL MED CNTR
CA	LOS ANGELES	CEDARS-SINAI MEDICAL CENTER
CA	LOS ANGELES	CHILDRENS HOSP OF LOS ANGELES
CA	LOS ANGELES	HOLLYWOOD PRESBYTERIAN M C
CA	LOS ANGELES	HOSPITAL OF THE GOOD SAMARITAN
CA	LOS ANGELES	KAISER FDN HOSP (CAD)
CA	LOS ANGELES	KAISER FDN HOSP (SUN)
CA	LOS ANGELES	LA COUNTY-USC MEDICAL CENTER
CA	LOS ANGELES	MARTIN LUTHER KING JR GEN HOSP
CA	LOS ANGELES	ORTHOPAEDIC HOSPITAL MED CNTR
CA	LOS ANGELES	QUEEN OF ANGELS MEDICAL CENTER
CA	LOS ANGELES	ST VINCENT MEDICAL CENTER
CA	LOS ANGELES	UCLA HOSPITAL & CLINICS
CA	LOS ANGELES	WHITE MEMORIAL MEDICAL CENTER
CA	LYNWOOD	ST FRANCIS MEDICAL CENTER
CA	MARTINEZ	VETERANS ADMIN MED CNTR
CA	MISSION VIEJO	MISSION COMMUNITY HOSPITAL
CA	MODESTO	MEMORIAL HOSPITALS ASSOCIATION
CA	MONTEBELLO	BEVERLY HOSPITAL
CA	MONTEREY PARK	GARFIELD MEDICAL CENTER
CA	NAPA	QUEEN OF THE VALLEY HOSPITAL
CA	NEWPORT BEACH	HOAG MEM HOSPITAL PRESBYTERIAN
CA	NORTHRIDGE	NORTHRIDGE HOSPITAL MED CNTR
CA	OAKLAND	NAVAL HOSPITAL
CA	OAKLAND	SAMUEL MERRITT HOSPITAL
CA	OCEANSIDE	TRI-CITY HOSPITAL
CA	ORANGE	CHILDRENS HSP OF ORANGE COUNTY
CA	ORANGE	ST JOSEPH HOSPITAL
CA	ORANGE	UNIV OF CALIF IRVINE MED CNTR
CA	OXNARD	ST JOHN'S HOSP REGL MED CNTR
CA	PALM SPRINGS	DESERT HOSPITAL
CA	PALO ALTO	PALO ALTO MEDICAL FOUNDATION

City	State	Hospital
CA	PALO ALTO	VETERANS ADMIN MED CNTR
CA	PANORAMA CITY	KAISER FDN HOSP (CAN)
CA	PANORAMA CITY	PANORAMA COMMUNITY HOSPITAL
CA	PASADENA	HUNTINGTON MEMORIAL HOSPITAL
CA	PASADENA	ST LUKE HOSPITAL OF PASADENA
CA	POMONA	POMONA VALLEY COMM HOSPITAL
CA	POWAY	POMERADO HOSPITAL
CA	RANCHO MIRAGE	EISENHOWER MEDICAL CENTER
CA	REDLANDS	REDLANDS COMMUNITY HOSPITAL
CA	REDONDO BEACH	SOUTH BAY HOSPITAL
CA	REDWOOD CITY	SEQUOIA HOSPITAL DISTRICT
CA	RIVERSIDE	PARKVIEW COMMUNITY HOSPITAL
CA	RIVERSIDE	RIVERSIDE COMMUNITY HOSPITAL
CA	RIVERSIDE	RIVERSIDE GEN HOSP-UN MED CNTR
CA	SACRAMENTO	MERCY HOSPITAL
CA	SACRAMENTO	SUTTER COMM HSPS OF SACRAMENTO
CA	SACRAMENTO	UNIV OF CALIF DAVIS MED CNTR
CA	SAN BERNARDINO	SAN BERNARDINO COMM HOSPITAL
CA	SAN BERNARDINO	SAN BERNARDINO COUNTY MED CNTR
CA	SAN BERNARDINO	ST BERNARDINE HOSPITAL
CA	SAN CLEMENTE	SAN CLEMENTE GENERAL HOSPITAL
CA	SAN DIEGO	CHILDRENS HOSP & HLTH CNTR
CA	SAN DIEGO	KAISER FDN HOSP (ZIO)
CA	SAN DIEGO	MERCY HOSPITAL & MED CNTR
CA	SAN DIEGO	NAVAL HOSPITAL
CA	SAN DIEGO	SHARP MEMORIAL HOSPITAL
CA	SAN DIEGO	UNIVERSITY HOSPITAL
CA	SAN DIMAS	SAN DIMAS COMMUNITY HOSPITAL
CA	SAN FRANCISCO	CHILDRENS HSP OF SAN FRANCISCO
CA	SAN FRANCISCO	FRENCH HOSPITAL/MEDICAL CENTER
CA	SAN FRANCISCO	LETTERMAN ARMY MEDICAL CENTER
CA	SAN FRANCISCO	MOUNT ZION HOSPITAL & MED CNTR
CA	SAN FRANCISCO	PRESBYTERIAN HOSPITAL
CA	SAN FRANCISCO	RALPH K DAVIS MEDICAL CENTER
CA	SAN FRANCISCO	SAN FRANCISCO GEN HOS M C
CA	SAN FRANCISCO	ST FRANCIS MEMORIAL HOSPITAL
CA	SAN FRANCISCO	ST LUKE'S HOSPITAL
CA	SAN FRANCISCO	ST MARY'S HOSPITAL & MED CNTR
CA	SAN FRANCISCO	UNIVERSITY OF CALIFORNIA, S.F.
CA	SAN GABRIEL	COMMUNITY HOSP OF SAN GABRIEL
CA	SAN JOSE	GOOD SAMARITAN HOSPITAL
CA	SAN JOSE	O'CONNOR HOSPITAL
CA	SAN JOSE	SAN JOSE HOSPITAL
CA	SAN JOSE	SANTA CLARA VALLEY MED CNTR
CA	SAN PABLO	BROOKSIDE HOSPITAL
CA	SAN PEDRO	SAN PEDRO PENINSULA HOSPITAL
CA	SANTA ANA	WESTERN MEDICAL CENTER
CA	SANTA BARBARA	GOLETA VALLEY COMM HOSPITAL
CA	SANTA BARBARA	SANTA BARBARA COTTAGE HOSPITAL
CA	SANTA BARBARA	ST FRANCIS HOSPITAL
CA	SANTA CRUZ	DOMINICAN SANTA CRUZ HOSPITAL
CA	SANTA MONICA	SANTA MONICA HOSPITAL MED CNTR
CA	SANTA MONICA	ST JOHN'S HOSPITAL & HLTH CNTR
CA	SOUTH LAGUNA	SOUTH COAST MEDICAL CENTER
CA	STOCKTON	DAMERON HOSPITAL ASSOCIATION
CA	STOCKTON	ST JOSEPH'S HOSPITAL
CA	TARZANA	MEDICAL CENTER OF TARZANA HOSP
CA	THOUSAND OAKS	LOS ROBLES REGIONAL MED CNTR
CA	TORRANCE	LA CNTY HARBOR-UCLA MED CNTR
CA	TORRANCE	LITTLE COMPANY OF MARY HOSP
CA	TORRANCE	TORRANCE MEM HOSPITAL MED CNTR
CA	TRAVIS AFB	DAVID GRANT USAF MED CNTR
CA	UPLAND	SAN ANTONIO COMMUNITY HOSPITAL
CA	VAN NUYS	VALLEY PRESBYTERIAN HOSPITAL
CA	VICTORVILLE	VICTOR VALLEY COMMUNITY HOSP
CA	VISALIA	KAWEAH DELTA DISTRICT HOSPITAL
CA	WALNUT CREEK	JOHN MUIR MEMORIAL HOSPITAL
CA	WEST COVINA	WEST COVINA HOSPITAL
CA	WHITTIER	PRESBYTERIAN INTERCOMM HOSP

City	State	Hospital
CO	AURORA	FITZSIMONS ARMY MEDICAL CENTER
CO	COLORADO SPRINGS	PENROSE HOSPITAL
CO	DENVER	PORTER MEMORIAL HOSPITAL
CO	DENVER	PRESBYTERIAN DENVER HOSPITAL
CO	DENVER	ROSE MEDICAL CENTER
CO	DENVER	SAINT JOSEPH HOSPITAL
CO	DENVER	SAINT LUKE'S HOSPITAL
CO	DENVER	ST ANTHONY HOSPITAL SYSTEMS
CO	DENVER	UNIVERSITY HOSP - UNIV OF CO
CO	DENVER	VETERANS ADMIN MED CNTR
CO	ENGLEWOOD	SWEDISH MEDICAL CENTER
CO	FORT CARSON	U S ARMY COMMUNITY HOSPITAL
CO	FORT COLLINS	POUDRE VALLEY HOSPITAL
CO	GREELEY	NORTH COLORADO MEDICAL CENTER
CO	LAKEWOOD	AMC·CANCER RESEARCH CNTR & HSP
CO	LONGMONT	LONGMONT UNITED HOSPITAL
CO	MONTROSE	MONTROSE MEMORIAL HOSPITAL
CO	PUEBLO	ST MARY-CORWIN HOSPITAL
CO	WHEAT RIDGE	LUTHERAN MEDICAL CENTER
CT	BRIDGEPORT	BRIDGEPORT HOSPITAL
CT	BRIDGEPORT	PARK CITY HOSPITAL
CT	BRIDGEPORT	ST VINCENT'S MEDICAL CENTER
CT	DANBURY	DANBURY HOSPITAL
CT	DERBY	GRIFFIN HOSPITAL
CT	FARMINGTON	U OF CT HLTH CTR/J DEMPSEY HSP
CT	GREENWICH	GREENWICH HOSPITAL ASSOCIATION
CT	HARTFORD	HARTFORD HOSPITAL
CT	HARTFORD	MOUNT SINAI HOSPITAL
CT	HARTFORD	SAINT FRANCIS HOSP & MED CNTR
CT	MERIDEN	MERIDEN-WALLINGFORD HOSPITAL
CT	MIDDLETOWN	MIDDLESEX MEMORIAL HOSPITAL
CT	NEW HAVEN	HOSPITAL OF ST RAPHAEL
CT	NEW HAVEN	YALE-NEW HAVEN HOSPITAL
CT	NORWALK	NORWALK HOSPITAL
CT	STAMFORD	ST JOSEPH HOSPITAL
CT	STAMFORD	STAMFORD HOSPITAL
CT	TORRINGTON	CHARLOTTE HUNGERFORD HOSPITAL
CT	WATERBURY	ST MARY'S HOSPITAL
CT	WATERBURY	WATERBURY HOSPITAL
DC	WASHINGTON	GEORGETOWN UNIVERSITY HOSPITAL
DC	WASHINGTON	GREATER SOUTHEAST COMM HOSP
DC	WASHINGTON	HOWARD UNIVERSITY HOSPITAL
DC	WASHINGTON	VETERANS ADMIN MED CNTR
DC	WASHINGTON	WALTER REED ARMY MEDICAL CNTR
DC	WASHINGTON	WASHINGTON HOSPITAL CENTER
DE	LEWES	BEEBE HOSPITAL OF SUSSEX CNTY
DE	WILMINGTON	ST FRANCIS HOSPITAL
DE	WILMINGTON	VETERANS ADMIN MED CNTR
DE	WILMINGTON	WILMINGTON MEDICAL CENTER
FL	DAYTONA BEACH	HALIFAX HOSPITAL MED CNTR
FL	DUNEDIN	MEASE HOSPITAL AND CLINIC
FL	GAINESVILLE	SHANDS HOSPITAL AT THE U OF FL
FL	JACKSONVILLE	NAVAL REGIONAL MEDICAL CENTER
FL	JACKSONVILLE	ST VINCENT'S MEDICAL CENTER
FL	JACKSONVILLE	UNIV HOSPITAL OF JACKSONVILLE
FL	LARGO	MEDICAL CENTER HOSPITAL
FL	MIAMI	CEDARS OF LEBANON HEALTH CNTR
FL	MIAMI	JACKSON MEMORIAL HOSPITAL
FL	MIAMI	NORTH SHORE MEDICAL CENTER
FL	MIAMI BEACH	MOUNT SINAI MEDICAL CENTER
FL	NAPLES	NAPLES COMMUNITY HOSPITAL

City	State	Hospital
FL	OCALA	MARION COMMUNITY HOSPITAL
FL	OCALA	MUNROE REGIONAL MEDICAL CENTER
FL	PENSACOLA	BAPTIST HOSPITAL
FL	PENSACOLA	NAVAL AEROSPACE & REGL MED CTR
FL	PENSACOLA	WEST FLORIDA HOSPITAL
FL	TALLAHASSEE	TALLAHASSEE MEM REGL MED CNTR
FL	TAMPA	ST JOSEPH'S HOSPITAL
FL	TAMPA	TAMPA GENERAL HOSPITAL
GA	ALBANY	PHOEBE PUTNEY MEM HOSPITAL
GA	AMERICUS	AMERICUS AND SUMTER CNTY HOSP
GA	ATLANTA	CRAWFORD W LONG MEM HOSPITAL
GA	ATLANTA	EMORY UNIVERSITY HOSPITAL
GA	ATLANTA	GEORGIA BAPTIST MEDICAL CENTER
GA	ATLANTA	GRADY MEMORIAL HOSPITAL
GA	ATLANTA	NORTHSIDE HOSPITAL
GA	ATLANTA	PIEDMONT HOSPITAL
GA	ATLANTA	ST JOSEPH'S HOSPITAL
GA	ATLANTA	WEST PACES FERRY HOSPITAL
GA	AUGUSTA	EUGENE TALMADGE MEML HOSPITAL
GA	AUSTELL	COBB GENERAL HOSPITAL
GA	COLUMBUS	THE MEDICAL CENTER
GA	DALTON	HAMILTON MEMORIAL HOSPITAL
GA	DECATUR	DEKALB GENERAL HOSPITAL
GA	DECATUR	VETERANS ADMIN MED CTR ATLANTA
GA	EAST POINT	SOUTH FULTON HOSPITAL
GA	FORT BENNING	MARTIN ARMY COMMUNITY HOSPITAL
GA	FORT GORDON	DWIGHT D EISENHOWER ARMY M C
GA	GAINESVILLE	NORTHEAST GEORGIA MED CNTR
GA	LA GRANGE	WEST GEORGIA MEDICAL CENTER
GA	MARIETTA	KENNESTONE HOSPITAL
GA	ROME	FLOYD MEDICAL CENTER
GA	SAVANNAH	MEMORIAL MEDICAL CENTER
GA	TOCCOA	STEPHENS COUNTY HOSPITAL
GA	VALDOSTA	SOUTH GEORGIA MEDICAL CENTER
HI	HONOLULU	KAISER FOUNDATION HOSPITAL
HI	HONOLULU	KUAKINI MEDICAL CENTER
HI	HONOLULU	QUEEN'S MEDICAL CENTER
HI	HONOLULU	ST FRANCIS HOSPITAL
HI	HONOLULU	STRAUB CLINIC AND HOSPITAL
HI	HONOLULU	TRIPLER ARMY MEDICAL CENTER
HI	LIHUE	G N WILCOX MEM HOS & HLTH CNTR
HI	WAILUKU	MAUI MEMORIAL HOSPITAL
HI	WAIMEA	KAUAI VETERANS MEM HOSPITAL
IA	DES MOINES	IOWA METHODIST MEDICAL CENTER
IA	DES MOINES	MERCY HOSPITAL MEDICAL CENTER
IA	DES MOINES	VETERANS ADMIN MED CNTR
IA	IOWA CITY	UNIV OF IOWA HOSPS & CLINICS
IA	MASON CITY	NORTH IOWA MEDICAL CENTER
IA	MASON CITY	ST JOSEPH MERCY HOSPITAL
IA	SIOUX CITY	MARIAN HEALTH CENTER
ID	BLACKFOOT	BINGHAM MEMORIAL HOSPITAL
ID	BOISE	ST ALPHONSUS REGL MED CNTR
ID	BOISE	ST LUKE'S HP/MTN STATES T INST
ID	BURLEY	CASSIA MEMORIAL HOS & MED CNTR
ID	LEWISTON	ST JOSEPH'S HOSPITAL
ID	NAMPA	MERCY MEDICAL CENTER
ID	POCATELLO	BANNOCK REGIONAL MEDICAL CTR
ID	TWIN FALLS	MAGIC VALLEY REGIONAL MED CNTR
IL	ARLINGTON HEIGHTS	NORTHWEST COMMUNITY HOSPITAL
IL	AURORA	COPLEY MEMORIAL HOSPITAL

City	State	Hospital
IL	AURORA	MERCY CNTR FOR HLTH CARE SERVS
IL	BERWYN	MACNEAL MEMORIAL HOSPITAL
IL	BLUE ISLAND	ST FRANCIS HOSPITAL
IL	CARBONDALE	MEMORIAL HOSP OF CARBONDALE
IL	CENTRALIA	ST MARY'S HOSPITAL
IL	CHAMPAIGN	BURNHAM HOSPITAL
IL	CHICAGO	BETHESDA HOSPITAL
IL	CHICAGO	CENTRAL COMMUNITY HOSPITAL
IL	CHICAGO	CHILDREN'S MEMORIAL HOSPITAL
IL	CHICAGO	COLUMBUS HOSPITAL
IL	CHICAGO	COOK COUNTY HOSPITAL
IL	CHICAGO	EDGEWATER HOSPITAL
IL	CHICAGO	FRANKLIN BOULEVARD COMM HOSP
IL	CHICAGO	HOLY CROSS HOSPITAL
IL	CHICAGO	ILLINOIS MASONIC MED CENTER
IL	CHICAGO	JACKSON PARK HOSPITAL
IL	CHICAGO	LOUIS A WEISS MEM HOSPITAL
IL	CHICAGO	MARY THOMPSON HOSPITAL
IL	CHICAGO	MERCY HOSPITAL AND MED CNTR
IL	CHICAGO	MICHAEL REESE HOSP & MED CNTR
IL	CHICAGO	MOUNT SINAI HOSPITAL MED CNTR
IL	CHICAGO	NORTHWESTERN MEMORIAL HOSPITAL
IL	CHICAGO	RAVENSWOOD HOSPITAL MED CNTR
IL	CHICAGO	RESURRECTION HOSPITAL
IL	CHICAGO	RUSH-PRESBY-ST LUKE'S MED CNTR
IL	CHICAGO	SOUTH CHICAGO COMM HOSPITAL
IL	CHICAGO	ST ANNE'S HOSPITAL
IL	CHICAGO	ST ELIZABETH'S HOSPITAL
IL	CHICAGO	ST JOSEPH HOSPITAL
IL	CHICAGO	ST MARY OF NAZARETH HOSP CNTR
IL	CHICAGO	SWEDISH COVENANT HOSPITAL
IL	CHICAGO	UNIV OF CHICAGO HSPS & CLINICS
IL	CHICAGO	UNIV OF ILLINOIS HOSPITAL
IL	CHICAGO	VETS ADMIN WEST SIDE MED CNTR
IL	CHICAGO HEIGHTS	ST JAMES HOSPITAL
IL	DANVILLE	LAKEVIEW MEDICAL CENTER
IL	DANVILLE	ST ELIZABETH HOSPITAL
IL	DE KALB	KISHWAUKEE COMMUNITY HOSPITAL
IL	DECATUR	DECATUR MEMORIAL HOSPITAL
IL	DES PLAINES	HOLY FAMILY HOSPITAL
IL	DIXON	KATHERINE SHAW BETHEA HOSPITAL
IL	EFFINGHAM	ST ANTHONY'S MEMORIAL HOSPITAL
IL	ELGIN	SAINT JOSEPH HOSPITAL
IL	ELGIN	SHERMAN HOSPITAL
IL	ELK GROVE VILLAGE	ALEXIAN BROTHERS MED CNTR
IL	ELMHURST	MEMORIAL HOSP OF DUPAGE COUNTY
IL	EVANSTON	EVANSTON HOSPITAL
IL	EVANSTON	ST FRANCIS HOSPITAL
IL	EVERGREEN PARK	LITTLE COMPANY OF MARY HOSP
IL	GALESBURG	ST MARY'S HOSPITAL
IL	GRANITE CITY	ST ELIZABETH MEDICAL CENTER
IL	GREAT LAKES	NAVAL REGIONAL MEDICAL CENTER
IL	HARVEY	INGALLS MEMORIAL HOSPITAL
IL	HIGHLAND PARK	HIGHLAND PARK HOSPITAL
IL	HINSDALE	HINSDALE HOSPITAL
IL	JOLIET	SAINT JOSEPH HOSPITAL
IL	KANKAKEE	ST MARY'S HOSPITAL OF KANKAKEE
IL	LAKE FOREST	LAKE FOREST HOSPITAL
IL	LIBERTYVILLE	CONDELL MEMORIAL HOSPITAL
IL	MACOMB	MCDONOUGH DISTRICT HOSPITAL
IL	MAYWOOD	F G MCGAW HOSP, LOYOLA UNIV MC
IL	MCHENRY	NORTHERN ILLINOIS MED CNTR
IL	MOLINE	LUTHERAN HOSPITAL
IL	NAPERVILLE	EDWARD HOSPITAL
IL	OAK LAWN	CHRIST HOSPITAL
IL	OAK PARK	WEST SUBURBAN HOSP MED CENTER
IL	OLNEY	RICHLAND MEMORIAL HOSPITAL
IL	PARK RIDGE	LUTHERAN GENERAL HOSPITAL
IL	PEORIA	METHODIST MED CNTR OF ILLINOIS
IL	PEORIA	ST FRANCIS HOSPITAL-MED CENTER

City	State	Hospital
IL	QUINCY	BLESSING HOSPITAL
IL	QUINCY	ST MARY HOSPITAL
IL	ROCKFORD	ROCKFORD MEMORIAL HOSPITAL
IL	ROCKFORD	ST ANTHONY HOSPITAL MED CTR
IL	ROCKFORD	SWEDISH-AMERICAN HOSPITAL
IL	SKOKIE	SKOKIE VALLEY COMM HOSPITAL
IL	SPRINGFIELD	MEMORIAL MEDICAL CENTER
IL	SPRINGFIELD	ST JOHN'S HOSPITAL
IL	STERLING	COMMUNITY GENERAL HOSPITAL
IL	URBANA	CARLE FOUNDATION HOSPITAL
IL	URBANA	MERCY HOSPITAL
IL	WAUKEGAN	ST THERESE HOSPITAL
IL	WINFIELD	CENTRAL DUPAGE HOSPITAL
IN	BLUFFTON	CAYLOR-NICKEL MEDICAL CENTER
IN	COLUMBUS	BARTHOLOMEW COUNTY HOSPITAL
IN	EAST CHICAGO	ST CATHERINE HOSP OF E CHIGAGO
IN	EVANSVILLE	DEACONESS HOSPITAL
IN	EVANSVILLE	ST MARY'S MEDICAL CENTER
IN	EVANSVILLE	WELBORN BAPTIST HOSPITAL
IN	GARY	METHODIST HOSPITAL OF GARY
IN	HAMMOND	ST MARGARET HOSPITAL
IN	INDIANAPOLIS	COMMUNITY HOSP OF INDIANAPOLIS
IN	INDIANAPOLIS	METHODIST HOSPITAL OF INDIANA
IN	INDIANAPOLIS	ST VINCENT HOSP & HLTH CNTR
IN	NEW ALBANY	MEMORIAL HOSPITAL
IN	SOUTH BEND	MEMORIAL HOSPITAL
IN	SOUTH BEND	ST JOSEPH'S MEDICAL CENTER
IN	TERRE HAUTE	TERRE HAUTE REGIONAL HOSPITAL
IN	TERRE HAUTE	UNION HOSPITAL
IN	VINCENNES	GOOD SAMARITAN HOSPITAL
LA	ALEXANDRIA	RAPIDES REGIONAL MED CTR
LA	ALEXANDRIA	ST FRANCES CABRINI HOSPITAL
LA	LAKE CHARLES	ST PATRICK HOS OF LAKE CHARLES
LA	NEW ORLEANS	CHARITY HOSPITAL OF LOUISIANA
LA	NEW ORLEANS	TOURO INFIRMARY
LA	NEW ORLEANS	VETERANS ADMIN MED CNTR
LA	SHREVEPORT	LSU MED CNTR-UNIVERSITY HOSP
LA	SHREVEPORT	VETERANS ADMIN MED CNTR
MA	ARLINGTON	CHOATE-SYMMES HEALTH SERVICES
MA	BEVERLY	BEVERLY HOSPITAL
MA	BOSTON	BOSTON CITY HOSPITAL
MA	BOSTON	BRIGHAM & WOMEN'S HOSPITAL
MA	BOSTON	CARNEY HOSPITAL
MA	BOSTON	CHILDREN'S HOSPITAL
MA	BOSTON	FAULKNER HOSPITAL
MA	BOSTON	MASSACHUSETTS GENERAL HOSPITAL
MA	BOSTON	NEW ENGLAND DEACONESS HOSPITAL
MA	BOSTON	ST ELIZABETH'S HOSP OF BOSTON
MA	BOSTON	UNIVERSITY HOSPITAL
MA	BROCKTON	BROCKTON HOSPITAL
MA	BROCKTON	CARDINAL CUSHING GEN HOSPITAL
MA	BURLINGTON	LAHEY CLINIC MEDICAL CENTER
MA	CAMBRIDGE	MOUNT AUBURN HOSPITAL
MA	CHELSEA	SOLDIERS HOME-QUIGLEY MEM HOSP
MA	CONCORD	EMERSON HOSPITAL
MA	DANVERS	HUNT MEMORIAL HOSPITAL
MA	FALL RIVER	ST ANNE'S HOSPITAL
MA	FRAMINGHAM	FRAMINGHAM UNION HOSPITAL
MA	HOLYOKE	HOLYOKE HOSPITAL
MA	HOLYOKE	PROVIDENCE HOSPITAL
MA	HYANNIS	CAPE COD HOSPITAL
MA	JAMAICA PLN, BOSTON	VETERANS ADMIN MED CNTR
MA	LOWELL	LOWELL GENERAL HOSPITAL
MA	LOWELL	ST JOHN'S HOSPITAL

City	State	Hospital
MA	LOWELL	ST JOSEPH'S HOSPITAL
MA	LYNN	LYNN HOSPITAL
MA	MEDFORD	LAWRENCE MEM HOSP OF MEDFORD
MA	MELROSE	MELROSE-WAKEFIELD HOSPITAL
MA	NATICK	LEONARD MORSE HOSPITAL
MA	NEEDHAM	GLOVER MEMORIAL HOSPITAL
MA	NEWTON LOWER FALLS	NEWTON-WELLESLEY HOSPITAL
MA	NORFOLK	SOUTHWOOD COMMUNITY HOSPITAL
MA	NORTH ADAMS	NORTH ADAMS REGIONAL HOSPITAL
MA	NORTHAMPTON	COOLEY DICKINSON HOSPITAL
MA	NORWOOD	NORWOOD HOSPITAL
MA	PITTSFIELD	BERKSHIRE MEDICAL CENTER
MA	PLYMOUTH	JORDAN HOSPITAL
MA	SALEM	SALEM HOSPITAL
MA	SOUTH WEYMOUTH	SOUTH SHORE HOSPITAL
MA	SPRINGFIELD	BAYSTATE MEDICAL CENTER
MA	SPRINGFIELD	MERCY HOSPITAL
MA	STONEHAM	NEW ENGLAND MEMORIAL HOSPITAL
MA	STOUGHTON	GODDARD MEMORIAL HOSPITAL
MA	WALTHAM	WALTHAM HOSPITAL
MA	WINCHESTER	WINCHESTER HOSPITAL
MA	WORCESTER	ST VINCENT HOSPITAL
MA	WORCESTER	WORCESTER MEMORIAL HOSPITAL
MD	ANNAPOLIS	ANNE ARUNDEL GENERAL HOSPITAL
MD	BALTIMORE	FRANKLIN SQUARE HOSPITAL
MD	BALTIMORE	JOHNS HOPKINS HOSPITAL
MD	BALTIMORE	SINAI HOSPITAL OF BALTIMORE
MD	BALTIMORE	SOUTH BALTIMORE GEN HOSPITAL
MD	BALTIMORE	UNIV OF MARYLAND HOSPITAL
MD	BETHESDA	NAVAL HOSPITAL
MD	CUMBERLAND	SACRED HEART HOSPITAL
MD	LEONARDTOWN	ST MARY'S HOSPITAL
MD	OLNEY	MONTGOMERY GENERAL HOSPITAL
MD	SALISBURY	'PENINSULA GENERAL HOS MED CNTR
MD	WASHINGTON, DC 20331	MALCOLM GROW USAF MED CNTR
ME	AUGUSTA	KENNEBEC VALLEY MEDICAL CENTER
ME	BANGOR	EASTERN MAINE MEDICAL CENTER
ME	LEWISTON	CENTRAL MAINE MEDICAL CENTER
ME	LEWISTON	ST MARY'S GENERAL HOSPITAL
ME	PORTLAND	MAINE MEDICAL CENTER
ME	PRESQUE ISLE	AROOSTOOK MEDICAL CENTER
ME	ROCKLAND	PENOBSCOT BAY MEDICAL CENTER
ME	RUMFORD	RUMFORD COMMUNITY HOSPITAL
ME	SKOWHEGAN	REDINGTON-FAIRVIEW GEN HOSP
ME	TOGUS	VETERANS ADMIN MED CNTR
ME	WATERVILLE	MID-MAINE MEDICAL CENTER
MI	ANN ARBOR	UNIVERSITY HOSPITAL
MI	BATTLE CREEK	LEILA HOSPITAL & HEALTH CENTER
MI	DEARBORN	OAKWOOD HOSPITAL
MI	DETROIT	DETROIT-MACOMB HOSPITAL CORPN
MI	DETROIT	HARPER-GRACE HOSPITAL
MI	DETROIT	HENRY FORD HOSPITAL
MI	FLINT	HURLEY MEDICAL CENTER
MI	FLINT	ST JOSEPH HOSPITAL
MI	GRAND RAPIDS	BLODGETT MEMORIAL MED CNTR
MI	GRAND RAPIDS	BUTTERWORTH HOSPITAL
MI	GRAND RAPIDS	FERGUSON HOSPITAL
MI	GRAND RAPIDS	ST MARY'S HOSPITAL
MI	KALAMAZOO	BORGESS MEDICAL CENTER
MI	KALAMAZOO	BRONSON METHODIST HOSPITAL
MI	LANSING	EDWARD W SPARROW HOSPITAL
MI	MARQUETTE	MARQUETTE GENERAL HOSPITAL

City	State	Hospital
MI	MENOMINEE	MENOMINEE COUNTY LLOYD HOSP
MI	MUSKEGON	HACKLEY HOSPITAL & MED CNTR
MI	ROCHESTER	CRITTENTON HOSPITAL
MI	ROYAL OAK	WILLIAM BEAUMONT HOSPITAL
MI	SAGINAW	ST MARY'S HOSPITAL
MI	SOUTHFIELD	PROVIDENCE HOSPITAL
MN	GRAND RAPIDS	ITASCA MEMORIAL HOSPITAL
MN	HIBBING	CENTRAL MESABI MEDICAL CENTER
MN	MANKATO	IMMANUEL-ST JOSEPH'S HOSPITAL
MN	MINNEAPOLIS	ABBOTT-NORTHWESTERN HOSPITAL
MN	MINNEAPOLIS	HENNEPIN COUNTY MEDICAL CENTER
MN	MINNEAPOLIS	METHODIST HOSPITAL
MN	MINNEAPOLIS	METROPOLITAN MEDICAL CENTER
MN	MINNEAPOLIS	MINNEAPOLIS CHILDREN'S M C
MN	MINNEAPOLIS	ST MARY'S HOSPITAL
MN	MINNEAPOLIS	VETERANS ADMIN MED CNTR
MN	MOORHEAD	ST ANSGAR HOSPITAL
MN	ROBBINSDALE	NORTH MEMORIAL MEDICAL CENTER
MN	ROCHESTER	MAYO CLINIC
MN	ST PAUL	ST PAUL-RAMSEY MEDICAL CENTER
MO	CAPE GIRARDEAU	SOUTHEAST MISSOURI HOSPITAL
MO	CAPE GIRARDEAU	ST FRANCIS MEDICAL CENTER
MO	COLUMBIA	BOONE HOSPITAL CENTER
MO	COLUMBIA	COLUMBIA REGIONAL HOSPITAL
MO	COLUMBIA	ELLIS FISCHEL STATE CANCER CTR
MO	COLUMBIA	UNIV OF MO HOSPITAL & CLINICS
MO	FORT LEONARD WOOD	GEN LEONARD WOOD ARMY HOSPITAL
MO	JEFFERSON CITY	MEMORIAL COMMUNITY HOSPITAL
MO	KANSAS CITY	BAPTIST MEDICAL CENTER
MO	KANSAS CITY	CHILDREN'S MERCY HOSPITAL
MO	KANSAS CITY	MENORAH MEDICAL CENTER
MO	KANSAS CITY	ST JOSEPH HOSP OF KANSAS CITY
MO	KANSAS CITY	ST LUKE'S HOSPITAL
MO	KANSAS CITY	TRINITY LUTHERAN HOSPITAL
MO	POPLAR BLUFF	DOCTORS REGIONAL MED CNTR
MO	SIKESTON	MISSOURI DELTA COMM HOSPITAL
MO	ST JOSEPH	METHODIST MEDICAL CENTER
MO	ST LOUIS	BARNES HOSPITAL
MO	ST LOUIS	CHRISTIAN HOSP N-EAST/N-WEST
MO	ST LOUIS	DEACONESS HOSPITAL
MO	ST LOUIS	INCARNATE WORD HOSPITAL
MO	ST LOUIS	JEWISH HOSPITAL OF ST. LOUIS
MO	ST LOUIS	ST ANTHONY'S MEDICAL CENTER
MO	ST LOUIS	ST JOHN'S MERCY MEDICAL CENTER
MO	ST LOUIS	ST LOUIS CHILDREN'S HOSPITAL
MO	ST LOUIS	ST MARY'S HEALTH CENTER
MO	ST LOUIS	VETERANS ADMIN MED CNTR-JC DIV
MS	BILOXI	BILOXI REGIONAL MEDICAL CENTER
MS	BILOXI	VETERANS ADMIN MED CNTR
MS	GULFPORT	MEMORIAL HOSPITAL AT GULFPORT
MS	HATTIESBURG	FORREST COUNTY GEN HOSPITAL
MS	HATTIESBURG	METHODIST HOSPITAL
MS	JACKSON	MISSISSIPPI BAPTIST MED CNTR
MS	JACKSON	UNIVERSITY HOSPITAL
MS	JACKSON	VETERANS ADMIN MED CNTR
MS	KEESLER AFB	USAF MEDICAL CENTER KEESLER
MS	OXFORD	OXFORD-LAFAYETTE CNTY HOSPITAL
MS	PASCAGOULA	SINGING RIVER HOSPITAL
MS	TUPELO	NORTH MISSISSIPPI MED CENTER
MS	VICKSBURG	MERCY REGIONAL MEDICAL CENTER
MT	GREAT FALLS	COLUMBUS HOSPITAL

City	State	Hospital
NC	CAMP LEJEUNE	NAVAL REGIONAL MEDICAL CENTER
NC	CHAPEL HILL	NORTH CAROLINA MEM HOSPITAL
NC	DURHAM	DUKE UNIVERSITY MEDICAL CENTER
NC	SHELBY	CLEVELAND MEMORIAL HOSPITAL
NC	VALDESE	VALDESE GENERAL HOSPITAL
NC	WINSTON-SALEM	NORTH CAROLINA BAPTIST HOSP
ND	FARGO	DAKOTA HOSPITAL AND CLINIC
ND	FARGO	ST JOHN'S HOSPITAL
ND	FARGO	ST LUKE'S HOSPITALS
ND	GRAND FORKS	THE UNITED HOSPITAL
ND	MINOT	ST JOSEPH'S HOSPITAL
ND	RUGBY	GOOD SAMARITAN HOSPITAL ASSN
ND	WILLISTON	MERCY HOSPITAL
NE	HASTINGS	MARY LANNING MEMORIAL HOSPITAL
NE	KEARNEY	GOOD SAMARITAN HOSPITAL
NE	LINCOLN	BRYAN MEMORIAL HOSPITAL
NE	LINCOLN	LINCOLN GENERAL HOSPITAL
NE	LINCOLN	ST ELIZABETH COMM HLTH CNTR
NE	LINCOLN	VETERANS ADMIN MED CNTR
NE	OMAHA	ARCHBISHOP BERGAN MERCY HOSP
NE	OMAHA	BISHOP CLARKSON MEML HOSPITAL
NE	OMAHA	IMMANUEL MEDICAL CENTER
NE	OMAHA	LUTHERAN MEDICAL CENTER
NE	OMAHA	NEBRASKA METHODIST HOSPITAL
NE	OMAHA	SAINT JOSEPH HOSPITAL
NE	OMAHA	UNIV OF NEBRASKA HOS & CLINICS
NH	CONCORD	CONCORD HOSPITAL
NH	DOVER	WENTWORTH-DOUGLASS HOSPITAL
NH	EXETER	EXETER HOSPITAL
NH	HANOVER	MARY HITCHCOCK MEM HOSPITAL
NH	KEENE	CHESHIRE HOSPITAL
NH	LACONIA	LAKES REGION GENERAL HOSPITAL
NH	LITTLETON	LITTLETON HOSPITAL
NH	MANCHESTER	CATHOLIC MEDICAL CENTER
NH	MANCHESTER	ELLIOT HOSPITAL
NH	PORTSMOUTH	PORTSMOUTH HOSPITAL
NH	ROCHESTER	FRISBIE MEMORIAL HOSPITAL
NJ	ATLANTIC CITY	ATLANTIC CITY MEDICAL CENTER
NJ	BELLEVILLE	CLARA MAASS MEDICAL CENTER
NJ	CAMDEN	WEST JERSEY HOSPITAL
NJ	DENVILLE	ST CLARE'S HOSPITAL
NJ	EAST ORANGE	VETERANS ADMIN MED CNTR
NJ	ELIZABETH	ELIZABETH GENERAL MED CENTER
NJ	ELIZABETH	ST ELIZABETH HOSPITAL
NJ	ENGLEWOOD	ENGLEWOOD HOSPITAL
NJ	HACKENSACK	HACKENSACK MEDICAL CENTER
NJ	HACKETTSTOWN	HACKETTSTOWN COMM HOSPITAL
NJ	LIVINGSTON	ST BARNABAS MEDICAL CENTER
NJ	LONG BRANCH	MONMOUTH MEDICAL CENTER
NJ	MONTCLAIR	MOUNTAINSIDE HOSPITAL
NJ	MORRISTOWN	MORRISTOWN MEMORIAL HOSPITAL
NJ	MOUNT HOLLY	BURLINGTON CNTY MEML HOSPITAL
NJ	NEPTUNE	JERSEY SHORE M C - FITKIN HOSP
NJ	NEW BRUNSWICK	MIDDLESEX GENL-UNIV HOSPITAL
NJ	NEWARK	NEWARK BETH ISRAEL MED CNTR
NJ	NEWARK	UNIVERSITY HOSPITAL
NJ	NEWTON	NEWTON MEMORIAL HOSPITAL
NJ	ORANGE	HOSPITAL CENTER AT ORANGE
NJ	PASSAIC	BETH ISRAEL HOSPITAL
NJ	PATERSON	ST JOSEPH'S HOSP & MED CNTR

City	State	Hospital
NJ	PHILLIPSBURG	WARREN HOSPITAL
NJ	PLAINFIELD	MUHLENBERG HOSPITAL
NJ	PRINCETON	MEDICAL CENTER AT PRINCETON
NJ	RED BANK	RIVERVIEW HOSPITAL
NJ	SOMERVILLE	SOMERSET MEDICAL CENTER
NJ	SUSSEX	WALLKILL VALLEY HOSPITAL
NJ	TEANECK	HOLY NAME HOSPITAL
NJ	TRENTON	ST FRANCIS MEDICAL CENTER
NJ	WESTWOOD	PASCACK VALLEY HOSPITAL
NM	ALBUQUERQUE	LOVELACE MEDICAL CENTER
NM	ALBUQUERQUE	ST JOSEPH HOSPITAL
NM	ALBUQUERQUE	UNIV OF NEW MEXICO HOSPITAL
NM	ALBUQUERQUE	VETERANS ADMIN MED CNTR
NV	LAS VEGAS	HUMANA HOSPITAL SUNRISE
NV	LAS VEGAS	SOUTHERN NEVADA MEM HOSPITAL
NY	ALBANY	VETERANS ADMIN MED CNTR
NY	AMITYVILLE	BRUNSWICK HOSPITAL CENTER
NY	BINGHAMTON	OUR LADY OF LOURDES MEM HOSP
NY	BRONX	BRONX-LEBANON HOSPITAL CENTER
NY	BRONX	MISERICORDIA HOSPITAL MED CNTR
NY	BRONX	VETERANS ADMIN MED CNTR
NY	BRONXVILLE	LAWRENCE HOSPITAL
NY	BROOKLYN	BROOKDALE HOSPITAL MED CNTR
NY	BROOKLYN	CALEDONIAN HOSPITAL
NY	BROOKLYN	CONEY ISLAND HOSPITAL
NY	BROOKLYN	DOWNSTATE MEDICAL CENTER
NY	BROOKLYN	INTERFAITH MEDICAL CENTER
NY	BROOKLYN	KINGS COUNTY HOSPITAL CENTER
NY	BROOKLYN	LONG ISLAND COLLEGE HOSPITAL
NY	BROOKLYN	LUTHERAN MEDICAL CENTER
NY	BROOKLYN	MAIMONIDES MEDICAL CENTER
NY	BROOKLYN	METHODIST HOSPITAL
NY	BROOKLYN	THE BROOKLYN HOSPITAL
NY	BROOKLYN	WYCKOFF HEIGHTS HOSPITAL
NY	BUFFALO	ROSWELL PARK MFM INSTITUTE
NY	BUFFALO	VETERANS ADMIN MED CNTR
NY	COBLESKILL	COMMUNITY HOSP SCHOHARIE CNTY
NY	COOPERSTOWN	MARY IMOGENE BASSETT HOSPITAL
NY	EAST MEADOW	NASSAU COUNTY MEDICAL CENTER
NY	ELMHURST	CITY HOSP CENTER AT ELMHURST
NY	ELMHURST	ST JOHNS QUEENS HOS DIV OF CMC
NY	ELMIRA	ARNOT-OGDEN MEMORIAL HOSPITAL
NY	ELMIRA	ST JOSEPH'S HOSPITAL
NY	FLUSHING	BOOTH MEMORIAL MEDICAL CENTER
NY	FLUSHING	FLUSHING HOSPITAL & MED CNTR
NY	FOREST HILLS	LA GUARDIA HOSPITAL
NY	GLEN COVE	THE COMMUNITY HOS AT GLEN COVE
NY	JAMAICA	JAMAICA HOSPITAL
NY	JAMAICA	MARY IMMACULATE HOS DIV OF CMC
NY	JAMAICA	QUEENS HOSPITAL CENTER
NY	JAMESTOWN	WOMAN'S CHRISTIAN ASSN HOSP
NY	JOHNSON CITY	CHARLES S WILSON MEM HOSPITAL
NY	MANHASSET	NORTH SHORE UNIV HOSPITAL
NY	MINEOLA	NASSAU HOSPITAL
NY	MOUNT KISCO	NORTHERN WESTCHESTER HOSP CNTR
NY	MOUNT VERNON	MOUNT VERNON HOSPITAL
NY	NEW HYDE PARK	LI JEWISH-HILLSIDE MED CNTR
NY	NEW ROCHELLE	NEW ROCHELLE HOSP MED CNTR
NY	NEW YORK	BELLEVUE HOSPITAL CENTER
NY	NEW YORK	BETH ISRAEL MEDICAL CENTER
NY	NEW YORK	CABRINI MEDICAL CENTER

City	State	Hospital
NY	NEW YORK	HARLEM HOSPITAL CENTER
NY	NEW YORK	MANHATTAN EE&T HOSPITAL
NY	NEW YORK	MEMORIAL HOSPITAL FOR CANCER
NY	NEW YORK	MONTEFIORE M C/MOSES DIV
NY	NEW YORK	NEW YORK INF/BEEKMAN DNTN HOSP
NY	NEW YORK	NEW YORK UNIV MEDICAL CENTER
NY	NEW YORK	PRESBYTERIAN HOSPITAL IN NYC
NY	NEW YORK	ST LUKE'S HOSPITAL DIVISION
NY	NEW YORK	ST VINCENT'S HOSP & MED CNTR
NY	NEW YORK	VETERANS ADMIN MED CNTR
NY	NYACK	NYACK HOSPITAL
NY	OCEANSIDE	SOUTH NASSAU COMMS HOSPITAL
NY	PATCHOGUE	BROOKHAVEN MEM HOSP MED CNTR
NY	PLAINVIEW	CENTRAL GENERAL HOSPITAL
NY	PORT JEFFERSON	JOHN T MATHER MEM HOSPITAL
NY	PORT JEFFERSON	ST CHARLES HOSPITAL
NY	PORT JERVIS	MERCY COMMUNITY HOSPITAL
NY	POUGHKEEPSIE	VASSAR BROTHERS HOSPITAL
NY	ROCHESTER	GENESEE HOSPITAL
NY	ROCHESTER	HIGHLAND HOSPITAL OF ROCHESTER
NY	ROCHESTER	PARK RIDGE HOSPITAL
NY	ROCHESTER	ROCHESTER GENERAL HOSPITAL
NY	ROCHESTER	ST MARY'S HOSPITAL
NY	ROCHESTER	STRONG MEMORIAL HOSPITAL
NY	ROCKVILLE CENTRE	MERCY HOSPITAL
NY	SARATOGA SPRINGS	SARATOGA HOSPITAL
NY	SCHENECTADY	ELLIS HOSPITAL
NY	STATEN ISLAND	BAYLEY SETON HOSPITAL
NY	STATEN ISLAND	DOCTORS' HOSP OF STATEN ISLAND
NY	STATEN ISLAND	ST VINCENT'S M C OF RICHMOND
NY	STATEN ISLAND	STATEN ISLAND HOSPITAL
NY	SYRACUSE	ST JOSEPH'S HOSPITAL HLTH CNTR
NY	SYRACUSE	UNIV HOSP OF UPSTATE MED CNTR
NY	TROY	SAMARITAN HOSPITAL
NY	VALLEY STREAM	FRANKLIN GENERAL HOSPITAL
NY	WALTON	DELAWARE VALLEY HOSPITAL
OH	AKRON	AKRON CITY HOSPITAL
OH	AKRON	AKRON GENERAL MEDICAL CENTER
OH	AKRON	ST THOMAS HOSPITAL MED CNTR
OH	BARBERTON	BARBERTON CITIZENS HOSPITAL
OH	CHARDON	GEAUGA COMMUNITY HOSPITAL
OH	CINCINNATI	BETHESDA HOSPITAL/OAK
OH	CINCINNATI	CHILDREN'S HOSPITAL MED CNTR
OH	CINCINNATI	GOOD SAMARITAN HOSPITAL
OH	CINCINNATI	JEWISH HOSPITAL OF CINCINNATI
OH	CINCINNATI	THE CHRIST HOSPITAL
OH	CINCINNATI	UNIV OF CINCINNATI HOSPITAL
OH	CLEVELAND	CLEVELAND CLINIC HOSPITAL
OH	CLEVELAND	DEACONESS HOSP OF CLEVELAND
OH	CLEVELAND	HURON ROAD HOSPITAL
OH	CLEVELAND	LUTHERAN MEDICAL CENTER
OH	CLEVELAND	ST ALEXIS HOSPITAL
OH	COLUMBUS	CHILDREN'S HOSPITAL
OH	COLUMBUS	GRANT HOSPITAL
OH	COLUMBUS	HAWKES HOSPITAL OF MT CARMEL
OH	COLUMBUS	OHIO STATE UNIV HOSPITALS
OH	COLUMBUS	RIVERSIDE METHODIST HOSPITAL
OH	DAYTON	GOOD SAMARITAN HOS & HLTH CNTR
OH	DAYTON	MIAMI VALLEY HOSPITAL
OH	DAYTON	ST ELIZABETH MEDICAL CENTER
OH	DOVER	UNION HOSPITAL ASSOCIATION
OH	ELYRIA	ELYRIA MEMORIAL HOSPITAL
OH	GALLIPOLIS	HOLZER MEDICAL CENTER
OH	KETTERING	KETTERING MEDICAL CENTER
OH	LORAIN	ST JOSEPH HOSPITAL

City	State	Hospital
OH	MARION	MARION GENERAL HOSPITAL
OH	MAYFIELD HEIGHTS	HILLCREST HOSPITAL
OH	MEDINA	MEDINA COMMUNITY HOSPITAL
OH	MIDDLEBURG HEIGHTS	SOUTHWEST GENERAL HOSPITAL
OH	OREGON	ST CHARLES HOSPITAL
OH	PARMA	PARMA COMMUNITY GEN HOSPITAL
OH	RAVENNA	ROBINSON MEMORIAL HOSPITAL
OH	SANDUSKY	GOOD SAMARITAN HOSPITAL
OH	SANDUSKY	PROVIDENCE HOSPITAL
OH	SPRINGFIELD	COMMUNITY HOSP OF SPRINGFIELD
OH	SPRINGFIELD	MERCY MEDICAL CENTER
OH	SYLVANIA	FLOWER HOSPITAL
OH	TOLEDO	MEDICAL COLLEGE OF OHIO HOSP
OH	TOLEDO	TOLEDO HOSPITAL
OH	URBANA	MERCY MEMORIAL HOSPITAL
OH	WRIGHT-PATTERSON AFB	USAF MED CTR WRIGHT-PATTERSON
OH	YOUNGSTOWN	ST ELIZABETH HOSPITAL MED CNTR
OH	YOUNGSTOWN	YOUNGSTOWN HOSPITAL ASSN
OK	ADA	VALLEY VIEW HOSPITAL
OK	BARTLESVILLE	JANE PHILLIPS EPISCOPAL-MEM MC
OK	CHICKASHA	GRADY MEMORIAL HOSPITAL
OK	MUSKOGEE	MUSKOGEE GENERAL HOSPITAL
OK	OKLAHOMA CITY	BAPTIST MEDICAL CENTER
OK	OKLAHOMA CITY	MERCY HEALTH CENTER
OK	OKLAHOMA CITY	OKLAHOMA CHILDREN'S MEM HOSP
OK	OKLAHOMA CITY	OKLAHOMA MEMORIAL HOSPITAL
OK	OKLAHOMA CITY	PRESBYTERIAN HOSPITAL
OK	OKLAHOMA CITY	SOUTH COMMUNITY HOSPITAL
OK	OKLAHOMA CITY	ST ANTHONY HOSPITAL
OK	OKMULGEE	OKMULGEE MEM HOSPITAL AUTH
OK	SHATTUCK	NEWMAN MEMORIAL HOSPITAL
OK	SHAWNEE	SHAWNEE MED CNTR HOSPITAL
OK	TULSA	HILLCREST MEDICAL CENTER
OK	TULSA	ST FRANCIS HOSPITAL
OK	TULSA	ST JOHN MEDICAL CENTER
OR	ALBANY	ALBANY GENERAL HOSPITAL
OR	CLACKAMAS	SUNNYSIDE MED CTR - KAISER FND
OR	CORVALLIS	GOOD SAMARITAN HOSPITAL
OR	EUGENE	SACRED HEART GENERAL HOSPITAL
OR	GRANTS PASS	JOSEPHINE MEMORIAL HOSPITAL
OR	KLAMATH FALLS	MERLE WEST MEDICAL CENTER
OR	LA GRANDE	GRANDE RONDE HOSPITAL
OR	MEDFORD	PROVIDENCE HOSPITAL
OR	MEDFORD	ROGUE VALLEY MEMORIAL HOSPITAL
OR	OREGON CITY	WILLAMETTE FALLS HOSPITAL
OR	PENDLETON	PENDLETON COMMUNITY HOSPITAL
OR	PENDLETON	ST ANTHONY HOSPITAL
OR	PORTLAND	BESS KAISER MEDICAL CENTER
OR	PORTLAND	EMANUEL HOSPITAL
OR	PORTLAND	GOOD SAMARITAN HOSP & MED CNTR
OR	PORTLAND	OREGON HEALTH SCIENCES UNIV
OR	PORTLAND	PHYSICIANS & SURGEONS HOSPITAL
OR	PORTLAND	PORTLAND ADVENTIST MED CNTR
OR	PORTLAND	PROVIDENCE MEDICAL CENTER
OR	PORTLAND	ST VINCENT HOSPITAL & MED CNTR
OR	PORTLAND	VETERANS ADMIN MED CNTR
OR	SALEM	SALEM HOSPITAL
OR	SPRINGFIELD	MCKENZIE-WILLAMETTE MEM HOSP
OR	TUALATIN	MERIDIAN PARK HOSPITAL
PA	ALLENTOWN	LEHIGH VALLEY HOSPITAL CENTER
PA	ALLENTOWN	SACRED HEART HOSPITAL

City	State	Hospital
PA	ALLENTOWN	THE ALLENTOWN HOSPITAL
PA	ALTOONA	ALTOONA HOSPITAL
PA	ALTOONA	MERCY HOSPITAL
PA	BETHLEHEM	ST LUKE'S HOSP OF BETHLEHEM
PA	BRYN MAWR	BRYN MAWR HOSPITAL
PA	DANVILLE	GEISINGER MEDICAL CENTER
PA	DREXEL HILL	DELAWARE COUNTY MEM HOSPITAL
PA	EASTON	EASTON HOSPITAL
PA	ERIE	HAMOT MEDICAL CENTER
PA	FRANKLIN	FRANKLIN REGIONAL MEDICAL CTR
PA	GREENSBURG	WESTMORELAND HOSPITAL
PA	GREENVILLE	GREENVILLE HOSPITAL
PA	HERSHEY	MILTON S HERSHEY MED CNTR
PA	JOHNSTOWN	CONEMAUGH VALLEY MEM HOSPITAL
PA	LANCASTER	LANCASTER GENERAL HOSPITAL
PA	LANCASTER	ST JOSEPH HOSPITAL
PA	LANSDALE	NORTH PENN HOSPITAL
PA	LATROBE	LATROBE AREA HOSPITAL
PA	LEWISTOWN	LEWISTOWN HOSPITAL
PA	NATRONA HEIGHTS	ALLEGHENY VALLEY HOSPITAL
PA	NEW CASTLE	JAMESON MEMORIAL HOSPITAL
PA	NORRISTOWN	MONTGOMERY HOSPITAL
PA	NORRISTOWN	SACRED HEART HOSPITAL
PA	PAOLI	PAOLI MEMORIAL HOSPITAL
PA	PHILADELPHIA	ALBERT EINSTEIN MC-NORTH DIV
PA	PHILADELPHIA	AMERICAN ONCOLOGIC HOSPITAL
PA	PHILADELPHIA	CHILDRENS HOSP OF PHILADELPHIA
PA	PHILADELPHIA	EPISCOPAL HOSPITAL
PA	PHILADELPHIA	GRADUATE HOSPITAL
PA	PHILADELPHIA	HAHNEMANN UNIVERSITY HOSPITAL
PA	PHILADELPHIA	HOSPITAL OF THE UNIV OF PENN
PA	PHILADELPHIA	JEANES HOSPITAL
PA	PHILADELPHIA	MERCY CATHOLIC MEDICAL CENTER
PA	PHILADELPHIA	MOUNT SINAI-DAROFF DIVISION OF
PA	PHILADELPHIA	PENNSYLVANIA HOSPITAL
PA	PHILADELPHIA	TEMPLE UNIVERSITY HOSPITAL
PA	PHILADELPHIA	THOMAS JEFFERSON UNIV HOSPITAL
PA	PITTSBURGH	ALLEGHENY GENERAL HOSPITAL
PA	PITTSBURGH	CHILDRENS HOSP OF PITTSBURGH
PA	PITTSBURGH	EYE AND EAR HOSP OF PITTSBURGH
PA	PITTSBURGH	MAGEE-WOMEN'S HOSPITAL
PA	PITTSBURGH	MERCY HOSPITAL OF PITTSBURGH
PA	PITTSBURGH	PRESBYTERIAN-UNIVERSITY HOSP
PA	PITTSBURGH	ST FRANCIS GENERAL HOSPITAL
PA	POTTSVILLE	POTTSVILLE HOSP & WARNE CLINIC
PA	QUAKERTOWN	QUAKERTOWN COMMUNITY HOSPITAL
PA	READING	READING HOSPITAL AND MED CNTR
PA	READING	SAINT JOSEPH HOSPITAL
PA	SAYRE	ROBERT PACKER HOSPITAL
PA	SCRANTON	MERCY HOSPITAL
PA	SCRANTON	MOSES TAYLOR HOSPITAL
PA	SELLERSVILLE	GRAND VIEW HOSPITAL
PA	STATE COLLEGE	CENTRE COMMUNITY HOSPITAL
PA	TUNKHANNOCK	TYLER MEMORIAL HOSPITAL
PA	WEST CHESTER	CHESTER COUNTY HOSPITAL
PA	WILKES-BARRE	VETERANS ADMIN MED CNTR
PA	WILLIAMSPORT	DIVINE PROVIDENCE HOSPITAL
PA	WILLIAMSPORT	WILLIAMSPORT HOSPITAL
PA	YORK	YORK HOSPITAL
PR	PONCE	CLINICA ONCOLOGICA GRILLASCA
PR	PONCE	HOSPITAL DAMAS
PR	SAN GERMAN	HOSPITAL DE LA CONCEPCION
PR	SAN JUAN	I GONZALEZ MARTINEZ ONCO HOSP
PR	SAN JUAN	UNIVERSITY HOSPITAL

City	State	Hospital
R I	NEWPORT	NAVAL REGIONAL MEDICAL CENTER
R I	PROVIDENCE	RHODE ISLAND HOSPITAL
R I	WARWICK	KENT COUNTY MEMORIAL HOSPITAL
SC	AIKEN	AIKEN COMMUNITY HOSPITAL
SC	ANDERSON	ANDERSON MEMORIAL HOSPITAL
SC	CHARLESTON	MEDICAL UNIV OF SOUTH CAROLINA
SC	COLUMBIA	BAPTIST MED CNTR AT COLUMBIA
SC	COLUMBIA	RICHLAND MEMORIAL HOSPITAL
SC	COLUMBIA	WM JENNINGS BRYAN DORN VETS HO
SC	FLORENCE	MCLEOD REGIONAL MEDICAL CENTER
SC	FORT JACKSON	MONCRIEF ARMY HOSPITAL
SC	GREENVILLE	GREENVILLE HOSPITAL SYSTEM
SC	GREENWOOD	SELF MEMORIAL HOSPITAL
SC	ORANGEBURG	ORANGEBURG REGIONAL HOSPITAL
SC	SPARTANBURG	SPARTANBURG GENERAL HOSPITAL
SD	ABERDEEN	ST LUKE'S HOSPITAL
SD	RAPID CITY	RAPID CITY REGIONAL HOSPITAL
SD	WATERTOWN	MEMORIAL MEDICAL CENTER
SD	WATERTOWN	ST ANN'S HOSPITAL
SD	YANKTON	SACRED HEART HOSPITAL
TN	BRISTOL	BRISTOL MEMORIAL HOSPITAL
TN	CHATTANOOGA	ERLANGER MEDICAL CENTER
TN	JOHNSON CITY	JOHNSON CITY MED CNTR HOSPITAL
TN	KINGSPORT	HOLSTON VALLEY HOSP & MED CNTR
TN	KNOXVILLE	EAST TENNESSEE BAPTIST HOSP
TN	KNOXVILLE	FORT SANDERS REGIONAL MED CNTR
TN	KNOXVILLE	UNIV OF TENNESSEE MEM HOSP
TN	MEMPHIS	BAPTIST MEMORIAL HOSPITAL
TN	MEMPHIS	METHODIST HOSPITALS OF MEMPHIS
TN	MEMPHIS	REGIONAL MED CTR AT MEMPHIS
TN	MEMPHIS	ST FRANCIS HOSPITAL
TN	MEMPHIS	ST JUDE CHILDREN'S RES HOSP
TN	MEMPHIS	UNIV OF TENN MEDICAL CENTER
TN	MILLINGTON	NAVAL REGL MED CNTR-MEMPHIS
TN	MOUNTAIN HOME	VETERANS ADMIN MED CNTR
TN	NASHVILLE	HUBBARD HOSP MEHARRY MED COLL
TN	NASHVILLE	METROPOLITAN NASHVILLE GEN HOS
TN	NASHVILLE	VANDERBILT UNIVERSITY HOSPITAL
TX	AMARILLO	HIGH PLAINS BAPTIST HOSPITAL
TX	AMARILLO	NORTHWEST TEXAS HOSPITAL
TX	AMARILLO	ST ANTHONY'S HOSPITAL
TX	AMARILLO	VETERANS ADMIN MED CNTR
TX	BIG SPRING	VETERANS ADMIN MED CNTR
TX	CARSWELL AFB	USAF REGIONAL HOSPITAL
TX	CORPUS CHRISTI	MEMORIAL MEDICAL CENTER
TX	CORPUS CHRISTI	NAVAL REGIONAL MEDICAL CENTER
TX	CORPUS CHRISTI	SPOHN HOSPITAL
TX	DALLAS	BAYLOR UNIV MEDICAL CENTER
TX	DALLAS	METHODIST HOSPITALS OF DALLAS
TX	DALLAS	PARKLAND MEM H/DALLAS CTY HOSP
TX	DALLAS	PRESBYTERIAN HOSP OF DALLAS
TX	DALLAS	ST PAUL HOSPITAL
TX	EL PASO	R E THOMASON GENERAL HOSPITAL
TX	EL PASO	WILLIAM BEAUMONT ARMY MED CNTR
TX	FORT SAM HOUSTON	BROOKE ARMY MEDICAL CENTER
TX	FORT WORTH	JOHN PETER SMITH HOSPITAL
TX	FORT WORTH	ST JOSEPH HOSPITAL
TX	GALVESTON	UNIV OF TEXAS MED BRANCH HOSPS

City	State	Hospital
TX	HARLINGEN	VALLEY BAPTIST MEDICAL CENTER
TX	HEREFORD	DEAF SMITH GENERAL HOSPITAL
TX	HOUSTON	BEN TAUB GENERAL HOSPITAL
TX	HOUSTON	M D ANDERSON HOS & TUMOR INST
TX	HOUSTON	PARK PLAZA HOSPITAL
TX	HOUSTON	ST JOSEPH HOSPITAL
TX	LACKLAND AFB	WILFORD HALL USAF MEDICAL CNTR
TX	LUBBOCK	HIGHLAND HOSPITAL
TX	LUBBOCK	METHODIST HOSPITAL
TX	MCALLEN	MCALLEN METHODIST HOSPITAL
TX	MIDLAND	MIDLAND MEMORIAL HOSPITAL
TX	ODESSA	MEDICAL CENTER HOSPITAL
TX	PLAINVIEW	CENTRAL PLAINS REGL HOSPITAL
TX	SAN ANGELO	ANGELO COMMUNITY HOSPITAL
TX	SAN ANTONIO	MEDICAL CENTER HOSPITAL
TX	SAN ANTONIO	SANTA ROSA MEDICAL CENTER
TX	SAN ANTONIO	SOUTHWEST TEXAS METHODIST HOSP
TX	TEMPLE	KING'S DAUGHTERS HOSPITAL
TX	TEMPLE	OLIN E TEAGUE VETERANS' CENTER
TX	TEMPLE	SCOTT AND WHITE MEM HOSPITAL
TX	TYLER	UNIV OF TEXAS HLTH CENTER
TX	WACO	HILLCREST BAPTIST MED CNTR
TX	WACO	PROVIDENCE HOSPITAL
TX	WHARTON	GULF COAST MEDICAL CENTER
UT	SALT LAKE CITY	HOLY CROSS HOSPITAL
UT	SALT LAKE CITY	LDS HOSPITAL
UT	SALT LAKE CITY	ST MARK'S HOSPITAL
UT	SALT LAKE CITY	UNIVERSITY OF UTAH HOSPITAL
UT	SALT LAKE CITY	VETERANS ADMIN MED CNTR
VA	ALEXANDRIA	THE ALEXANDRIA HOSPITAL
VA	ARLINGTON	ARLINGTON HOSPITAL
VA	ARLINGTON	NORTHERN VIRGINIA DOCTORS HOSP
VA	BIG STONE GAP	LONESOME PINE HOSPITAL
VA	CHARLOTTESVILLE	UNIV OF VIRGINIA HOSPITAL
VA	CHESAPEAKE	CHESAPEAKE GENERAL HOSPITAL
VA	DANVILLE	MEMORIAL HOSPITAL
VA	FAIRFAX	COMMONWEALTH HOSPITAL
VA	FALLS CHURCH	FAIRFAX HOSPITAL
VA	FREDERICKSBURG	MARY WASHINGTON HOSPITAL
VA	HAMPTON	VETERANS ADMIN MED CNTR
VA	HARRISONBURG	ROCKINGHAM MEMORIAL HOSPITAL
VA	LEESBURG	LOUDOUN MEMORIAL HOSPITAL
VA	LOW MOOR	ALLEGHANY REGIONAL HOSPITAL
VA	LYNCHBURG	LYNCHBURG GEN-MARSHALL LODGE H
VA	LYNCHBURG	VIRGINIA BAPTIST HOSPITAL
VA	NEWPORT NEWS	RIVERSIDE HOSPITAL
VA	NORFOLK	DEPAUL HOSPITAL
VA	NORFOLK	NORFOLK GENERAL HOSPITAL
VA	PORTSMOUTH	NAVAL REGIONAL MEDICAL CENTER
VA	RICHMOND	MED COLLEGE OF VIRGINIA HOSPS
VA	RICHMOND	ST LUKE'S HOSPITAL
VA	RICHMOND	ST MARY'S HOSPITAL
VA	ROANOKE	COMM HOSP OF ROANOKE VALLEY
VA	ROANOKE	ROANOKE MEMORIAL HOSPITALS
VA	SALEM	LEWIS-GALE HOSPITAL
VA	SALEM	VETERANS ADMIN MED CNTR
VA	WINCHESTER	WINCHESTER MEMORIAL HOSPITAL
VT	BENNINGTON	SOUTHWESTERN VERMONT MED CNTR
VT	BURLINGTON	MEDICAL CENTER HOSP OF VERMONT
VT	RANDOLPH	GIFFORD MEMORIAL HOSPITAL
VT	RUTLAND	RUTLAND REGL MEDICAL CENTER

City	State	Hospital
WA	ABERDEEN	GRAYS HARBOR COMM HOSPITAL
WA	ABERDEEN	ST JOSEPH HOSPITAL
WA	ANACORTES	ISLAND HOSPITAL
WA	BELLEVUE	OVERLAKE HOSPITAL
WA	BELLINGHAM	ST JOSEPH HOSPITAL
WA	BELLINGHAM	ST LUKE'S GENERAL HOSPITAL
WA	BREMERTON	HARRISON MEMORIAL HOSPITAL
WA	BREMERTON	NAVAL HOSPITAL
WA	COUPEVILLE	WHIDBEY GENERAL HOSPITAL
WA	EDMONDS	STEVENS MEMORIAL HOSPITAL
WA	EVERETT	GENERAL HOSPITAL OF EVERETT
WA	EVERETT	PROVIDENCE HOSPITAL
WA	KENNEWICK	KENNEWICK GENERAL HOSPITAL
WA	KIRKLAND	EVERGREEN GENERAL HOSPITAL
WA	LONGVIEW	MONTICELLO MEDICAL CENTER
WA	LONGVIEW	ST JOHN'S HOSPITAL
WA	MOUNT VERNON	SKAGIT VALLEY HOSPITAL
WA	OLYMPIA	ST PETER HOSPITAL
WA	PASCO	OUR LADY OF LOURDES HOSPITAL
WA	SEATTLE	CHILDRENS ORTHO HOS & MED CNTR
WA	SEATTLE	GROUP HEALTH COOP CENTRAL HOSP
WA	SEATTLE	NORTHWEST HOSPITAL
WA	SEATTLE	PROVIDENCE MEDICAL CENTER
WA	SEATTLE	SWEDISH HOSP MEDICAL CENTER
WA	SEATTLE	VIRGINIA MASON HOSPITAL
WA	SEDRO WOOLLEY	UNITED GENERAL HOSPITAL
WA	SPOKANE	DEACONESS HOSPITAL
WA	SPOKANE	SACRED HEART MEDICAL CENTER
WA	TACOMA	MADIGAN ARMY MEDICAL CENTER
WA	TACOMA	TACOMA GENERAL HOSPITAL
WA	VANCOUVER	SOUTHWEST WASHINGTON HOSPITALS
WA	WALLA WALLA	ST MARY COMMUNITY HOSPITAL
WA	WALLA WALLA	WALLA WALLA GENERAL HOSPITAL
WA	WENATCHEE	WENATCHEE VALLEY CLINIC
WA	YAKIMA	ST ELIZABETH HOSPITAL
WA	YAKIMA	YAKIMA VALLEY MEM HOSPITAL
WI	CUDAHY	TRINITY MEMORIAL HOSPITAL
WI	EAU CLAIRE	LUTHER HOSPITAL
WI	EAU CLAIRE	SACRED HEART HOSPITAL
WI	FOND DU LAC	ST AGNES HOSPITAL
WI	GREEN BAY	ST VINCENT HOSPITAL
WI	JANESVILLE	MERCY HOSPITAL
WI	LA CROSSE	LA CROSSE LUTHERAN HOSPITAL
WI	LA CROSSE	ST FRANCIS MEDICAL CENTER
WI	MADISON	MADISON GENERAL HOSPITAL
WI	MARINETTE	MARINETTE GENERAL HOSPITAL
WI	MARSHFIELD	MARSHFIELD CLNC/ST JOSEPH'S H
WI	MILWAUKEE	COLUMBIA HOSPITAL
WI	MILWAUKEE	GOOD SAM MC-DEACONESS H CAMPUS
WI	MILWAUKEE	MILWAUKEE CNTY MED COMPLEX
WI	MILWAUKEE	MOUNT SINAI MEDICAL CENTER
WI	MILWAUKEE	ST FRANCIS HOSPITAL
WI	MILWAUKEE	ST JOSEPH'S HOSPITAL
WI	MILWAUKEE	ST LUKE'S HOSPITAL
WI	MILWAUKEE	ST MARY'S HOSPITAL
WI	MILWAUKEE	ST MICHAEL HOSPITAL
WI	MILWAUKEE	VETERANS ADM MEDICAL CENTER
WI	MONROE	ST CLARE HOSPITAL OF MONROE
WI	OSHKOSH	MERCY MEDICAL CENTER
WI	WAUSAU	WAUSAU HOSPITAL CENTER
WI	WEST ALLIS	WEST ALLIS MEMORIAL HOSPITAL
WV	CHARLESTON	CHARLESTON AREA MEDICAL CENTER
WV	CLARKSBURG	LOUIS A JOHNSON VA MED CNTR

City	State	Hospital
WV	ELKINS	DAVIS MEMORIAL HOSPITAL
WV	ELKINS	MEMORIAL GENERAL HOSP ASSOC
WV	HUNTINGTON	SAINT MARY'S HOSPITAL
WV	HUNTINGTON	VETERANS ADMIN MED CNTR
WV	MONTGOMERY	MONTGOMERY GENERAL HOSPITAL
WV	MORGANTOWN	WEST VIRGINIA UNIV HOSPITAL
WV	PARKERSBURG	CAMDEN-CLARK MEMORIAL HOSPITAL
WV	WHEELING	OHIO VALLEY MEDICAL CENTER
WY	CHEYENNE	DE PAUL HOSPITAL
WY	CHEYENNE	MEMORIAL HOSP OF LARAMIE CNTY

Glossary

This brief glossary consists mainly of terms whose meanings are sometimes difficult to remember. It is not intended to be a complete listing of the medical terminology used in this book but instead a reminder of the meaning of the more pertinent terms. Included also are a few common terms that might be encountered when reading other books on cancer. This glossary should not preclude use of a dictionary, because definitions are given only in the context of cancer biology.

Actin: Protein subunit of microfilaments.
Actinomycin D: An inhibitor of RNA synthesis.
Adenoma: Benign tumor of glandular tissue.
Alkylating agents: A group of compounds that chemically modify DNA; some are carcinogens and some are antitumor agents.
Anaplastic: Without form.
Antibiotic: Antibacterial agent produced by microorganisms; some antibiotics have anticancer activity.
Antibody: A protein produced in animals in response to a specific antigen and capable of binding that antigen.
Antigen: Any substance capable of stimulating production of specific antibodies.
Aneuploid: Having an abnormal chromosome number.
Axillary lymph nodes: Lymph nodes in the arm pits.
Azo dyes: A group of compounds that are often carcinogenic.
B-cells: Lymphocytes involved in production of antibodies.
Basal cell carcinoma: Common form of skin cancer that forms in the innermost skin layer.
BCG (Bacillus Calmette-Guerin): Weakened form of tuberculosis bacterium used to stimulate the immune system.
Benign tumor: Slow growing, nonspreading growth that usually does not harm the host.

Biopsy: Removal of small tissue sample from the body for microscopic examination.

Bone marrow transplant: Replacement of diseased bone marrow killed by radiation and chemicals with healthy bone marrow from a compatible donor.

Bronchoscopy: Direct viewing of the lung by fiber optics.

Burkitt's lymphoma: A lymphoid cancer associated with Epstein-Barr virus.

Cancer: A group of diseases characterized by uncontrolled cell growth and spread.

Carcinogen: A cancer-causing agent.

Carcinogenesis: Induction of cancer cell formation.

Carcinoma: Cancer derived from epithelial tissue.

Carcinoma in situ: Cancer that is confined to the tissue of origin and has not yet spread.

Cellular immunity: Direct attack by lymphocytes on foreign cells.

Cervix: Neck of the uterus.

Chemotherapy: Treatment of disease with drugs.

Colonoscopy: Direct visual examination of the large intestine using a lighted, flexible tube.

Contact inhibition: The inhibition of growth or movement of cells upon contact with other cells.

Dysplasia: Abnormal organization of cells and tissues.

Endometrium: Lining of the uterus.

Endotoxin: Immunotherapeutic agent isolated from cell walls of certain bacteria.

Epidemiology: Study of the incidence, distribution, environmental causes, and control of disease in population groups.

Epithelium: Surface covering of an organ or tissue.

Epstein-Barr virus: A virus associated with Burkitt's lymphoma and infectious mononucleosis.

Etiology: Study of the causes of diseases.

Gamma ray: Electromagnetic radiation emitted by some radioactive atoms.

Gene: A sequence of DNA that codes for a polypeptide (protein) chain; a unit of hereditary information in chromosomes.

Hodgkin's disease: A type of lymphoid cancer.

Hyperplasia: Abnormal proliferation of cells in a tissue.

Hysterectomy: Surgical removal of the uterus.

Immunotherapy: Treatment of disease by stimulating the body's immune system to fight off the disease.

Initiation: First step in a two-step process involved in cancer induction.

Interferon: A protein made by cells to inhibit virus multiplication; stimulates NK (killer) cells to destroy cancer cells.

Invasion: Growth of cancer by expanding and cell movements into neighboring tissues.

Karyotype: Chromosome size, shape, and number of a particular cell.

Lectin: Carbohydrate-binding protein.

Leukemia: Cancer of the blood-forming tissue in which white blood cell number increases greatly.

Leukocyte: A white blood cell.

Lymph node: A gland-like body involved in the immune system.
Lymphocyte: A white blood cell involved in the immune response.
Lymphoma: Cancer of the lymph nodes.
Lymphosarcoma: Cancer of lymphoid tissue.
Lysosome: Cytoplasmic body containing degradative enzymes.
Malignant tumor: A cancer; an abnormal growth that spreads and can destroy the host.
Mammography: X-ray technique for locating breast abnormalities.
Mastectomy: Surgical removal of a breast. Radical mastectomy involves removal of the breast, muscle tissue, and lymph nodes in the armpit. Simple mastectomy involves removal of the breast only.
Melanoma: Highly malignant cancer of the pigment-forming cells.
Metastasis: Development of secondary cancers by distant spread of cells from primary cancers.
Microfilament: Rod-like element composed of the protein actin.
Microtubule: Cylindrical unit composed of globular subunits of the protein tubulin.
Mutation: Heritable change in DNA.
Neoplasia: Process of forming new growth; often used to mean formation of cancer.
Neoplasm: Abnormal growth of cells; often used to mean a malignant tumor.
Oncogene: A gene whose gene product is involved in induction of cancer.
Oncogenic: Cancer-causing.
Oncology: The study of cancer.
Palliative treatment: Relieving symptoms of a disease but not directly curing the disease.
Palpation: Use of fingers to feel the body for the purpose of diagnosis of abnormalities.
Pap test: Microscopic examination of secretions from the vagina to diagnose cervical cellular abnormalities.
Plasma cell: A mature antibody-secreting B lymphocyte.
Polyoma virus: DNA virus that induces cancer in some animals.
Polyp: Tissue outgrowth projecting into the cavity of an organ or the bodyl.
Polyposis: Condition of having many polyps in an organ or structure.
Primary tumor: Tumor resulting from transformation of normal cells into tumor cells.
Prognosis: The prospects for the future or outcome of a disease.
Promotion: The second step in the two-step process of development of some cancers.
Protease: A protein-degrading enzyme.
Protooncogene: A gene that can be activated to cause cancer; usually, the normal counterpart of an oncogene.
Radiation therapy: Cancer treatment with radiation that kills cells.
Remission: Disappearance of the signs of a disease.
Retinoblastoma: Cancer of the retina of the eye.
Retrovirus: A virus in whose life cycle RNA is converted to DNA.
Reverse transcriptase: An enzyme that catalyzes the synthesis of DNA using RNA as a template.
Rous sarcoma virus: A retrovirus that can cause cancer in chickens.

Sarcoma: Cancer derived from connective tissue and muscle.

Simian virus 40 (SV40): A DNA tumor virus.

Squamous cell carcinoma: Cancer of flat surface cells.

T cell: Lymphocyte that plays a major role in cellular immunity.

Thermography: Measurement of surface temperature of body regions to detect diseases such as breast cancer.

Transformation: Change of normal cells into more abnormal cells with characteristics similar to cancer cells.

Tumor: Abnormal swelling or enlarged mass that is either benign or malignant.

Tumor-specific (-associated) antigen: Antigen found primarily on or in tumor cells.

Wilm's tumor: Embryonic kidney tumor primarily affecting young children.

Xeroradiography: An x-ray photographic technique that is used to detect breast cancer.

X rays: Electromagnetic radiation of extremely short wavelength.

Index